Anxiety Disorders

Anxiety Disorders

Psychological Assessment and Treatment

Vimala Veeraraghavan
Shalini Singh

Sage Publications
New Delhi • Thousand Oaks • London

BS

First published in 2002 by

Sage Publications India Pvt Ltd
M-32 Market, Greater Kailash-I
New Delhi 110 048

Sage Publications Inc.
2455 Teller Road
Thousand Oaks, California 91320

Sage Publications Ltd
6 Bonhill Street
London EC2A 4PU

Published by Tejeshwar Singh for Sage Publications India Pvt Ltd, type-set in 10.5 pt Garamond by Line Arts, Pondicherry and printed at Chaman Enterprises, Delhi.

Library of Congress Cataloging-in-Publication Data

Veeraraghavan, Vimala, 1936–
   Anxiety disorders: psychological assessment and treatment/Vimala Veeraraghavan, Shalini Singh.
     p. cm.
  Includes bibliographical references and index.
   1. Anxiety—Treatment. I. Singh, Shalini, 1970– II. Title.
   RC531 V445 616.85'223—dc21   2002   2001048290

ISBN: 0–7619–9558–7 (US-Pb)   81–7829–065–0 (India-Pb)
         0–7619–9615–X (US-Hb)   81–7829–085–5 (India-Hb)

Sage Production Team: Urmila Kalra, Bhanu Pratap Sharma, Mathew P.J. and Santosh Rawat

10/10/03

contents

Preface

In everyday contexts, anxiety is a term used to describe uncomfortable and unpleasant feelings that an individual experiences when in stressful or fearful situations. As an emotion, it is characterized primarily by feelings of dread, worry, fear and apprehension. Anxiety is experienced by every individual at some point or other in his/her life, for example, while making a presentation, appearing for an interview, waiting for test results, facing the boss, walking through a dark, unfamiliar street, and so on. In addition, anxiety may be triggered in response to specific situations, people or events, as well as in anticipation of an event.

The experience of anxiety can best be understood on a continuum from a normal, adaptive response, to the demands of a hectic life full of pressures, deadlines and stress, to a more severe form which disrupts a person's daily functioning. Anxious individuals commonly report feeling out of control. The subjective experience of anxiety may be accompanied by physical symptoms such as an increased heart and respiration rate, desire to urinate, sweating, and muscular tension. The associated unpleasantness may be so distressing that it could lead the individual to avoid the anxiety-arousing situation and hence the fear associated with it.

Worry, fear and anxiety are encountered commonly in therapeutic settings but anxiety that is severe, persistent and irrational requires professional intervention. In clinical settings, anxiety disorders refer to states where severe free-floating anxiety is the main feature. *Diagnostic and Statistical Manual of Mental Disorders*, 4/e (DSM IV) includes agoraphobia (with or without panic disorder), panic disorder, specific phobia, social phobia, post-traumatic stress disorder, acute stress disorder, obsessive-compulsive disorder, generalized anxiety disorder, anxiety due to a general medical condition, substance-induced anxiety and anxiety not otherwise specified. In a clinical setup, anxiety disorders may present themselves exclusively or in co-morbidity.

Over the years, there have been innumerable attempts to deal with these disorders. At different times in history, different types of treatments have been tried out with mixed success. While psychoanalytical and other psychotherapies claimed success in treating the anxiety disorders, in recent years behavior therapies appear to have been more successful. It may be mentioned here that even cognitive therapies, rational emotive therapy and many indigenous therapies such as yoga and meditation have been demonstrated to be effective in treating these disorders successfully.

While there are books on abnormal psychology, clinical psychology, and psychiatry covering the Indian scenario, there is an almost negligible number of books that deal with diagnosis, assessment and treatment of anxiety disorders with actual case studies and case illustrations. Books from the western world provide tried and tested techniques in handling anxiety disorders but use case studies in the western context. The present book attempts to remove this lacuna. While it does not rely on any particular school of thought, it does emphasize the relevance and importance of an eclectic or holistic approach in the treatment of anxiety disorders.

The book is structured as follows: Chapter 1 provides a brief overview, including concepts, definitions and the various manifestations of anxiety disorders. The etiological perspectives of anxiety disorders from different schools of thought have been presented in Chapter 2 to help readers get an overall view of the possible causes. The dictum that effective treatment requires an accurate diagnosis is stressed, since successful and effective treatment depends on a thorough assessment. Chapter 3 highlights the techniques and tools required to make an adequate assessment. An important issue that has been tackled in the book is how to effectively treat anxiety disorders and help the patient become asymptomatic. Presented in Chapter 4 are some important psychological treatment techniques used exclusively as well as in combination with other therapies. As is obvious, each patient is unique concerning his/her personality, family constellation, interactional process, social support and other related aspects. This naturally demands that the intervention program combine different therapies. In some cases, the individual approach has to be emphasized, and in others, family therapy. Combining therapies to suit the individual's needs, symptoms and problems is known as the multimodal approach and has been tried out in the treatment of anxiety disorders. Cases presented in this chapter clearly show the differential combination of supportive therapy, behavior modification, family therapy, cognitive therapy, etc., and in differing ways depending on the needs of individuals in each of the cases presented. Each case also contains the procedure by which the differential diagnosis was arrived at and the manner in which treatment strategies were planned and carried out.

While therapists may be effective and the results in the desired direction, therapist and trainees often come across difficulties during the course of the session, resulting, for example, in dropouts, blind alleys, unresolved transference and counter-transference. Chapter 5 presents some of the difficulties faced by the therapist and offers solutions. The book also includes a handy Appendix which provides the reader with step-by-step procedures of the more commonly used techniques in clinical settings.

The authors have attempted to bring to the fore the importance of an eclectic approach towards therapy and have, in the process, demonstrated the nature of combining therapies even though one may subscribe to a particular school of thought such as the Psychoanalytical or Learning School. In the present context, especially in India, patients often demand quick and lasting results and many do not want to experience the side effects of drugs. Biofeedback, Yoga, Reiki, Pranic healing, meditation and many indigenous treatments are used by patients in their search for alternatives to drug therapies. The use of psychological treatment with its refined, objective and individualized approach which uses a combination of therapies to suit the patient, could fill the void left by the several of the earlier schools which followed a single approach.

There is still considerable scope for improvement in the methods of psychological treatment and, as one glances at the literature available, it is heartening to note that many new therapies are being developed and used. What is required for effective treatment of anxiety disorders is an open approach by the therapist to include different forms of therapies with the main goal of returning the patient to normalcy. The book has made a contribution towards this end and it is hoped that therapists may find it possible to try out the steps given in various therapies.

Nov. 2001   **Authors**

1
Overview of Anxiety Disorders

overview

Children, adolescents, and adults experience anxiety in different forms; this is visible in some and can be inferred in others from their physiological and psychological responses. Anxiety also varies in frequency and intensity in different persons, often in response to the same stimulus. While anxiety may drive some towards positive action, in others it may lead to non-action, almost paralyzing them by its overwhelming presence. A certain amount of anxiety is considered essential to get a person to perform at his/her highest levels of efficiency and productivity, but beyond a point it adversely affects both these. Thus, anxiety may be a positive or negative condition in a person though it generally originates as a symptom of psychiatric disorders.

conceptualization of anxiety

Anxiety is often a diffuse, unpleasant and uncomfortable feeling of apprehension, accompanied by one or more bodily sensations that characteristically recur in the same manner in the person. It is an alerting signal that warns an individual of imminent danger and enables him to take measures to deal with it. Anxiety and fear may exist simultaneously or follow each other. Anxiety or fear-arousing stimulus may be internal, external, immediate or future, definite or vague, conflictual or non-conflictual in nature. One can, however, differentiate anxiety from fear, in that, in fear no conflict is involved and the threat is known. According to *Hallam (1992)*, anxiety is a word used in everyday conversation, and refers to a complex relationship between a person and his situation. It may refer to (*a*) the behavior of a person (*b*) appraisal of the responses and their effect (*c*) his intentions towards a situation and (*d*) his evaluation of the resources available for dealing with it.

There is no single set of biological or psychological processes that define anxiety and it is also not possible to consider anxiety purely in objective terms, that is, as a state of the organism. This is because the concept of anxiety is used differently by different people, and even the same person may use anxiety differently on different occasions.

There are broadly two ways of conceptualizing anxiety: behavioral and non-behavioral. When anxiety is defined from a behavioral perspective, it is taken as a set of responses involving a combination of cognitive and physiological responses, as well as the external stimuli and related situations. This physiological state of anxiety is associated with increased activation of the sympathetic pathways of the autonomic nervous system and prepares the body for vigorous muscular activity. It usually includes (*a*) accelerated heart rate and an increase in the blood volume being pumped with each beat (*b*) sweating, which triggers a rise in skin conductivity (*c*) rapid respiration (*d*) inhibition of salivation, stomach contractions, digestive secretions and (*e*) dilation of pupils and inhibition of tear glands. These reactions are often expressed by the patient as "trembling", "pounding heart", "knot in the stomach", and so on. They are accompanied by a rise in muscular tension throughout the body resulting in fatigue.

In addition to the foregoing physiological or somatic patterning that indicates the anxiety level in a patient, it also accounts for the following interpretations: (*a*) subjective interpretations of these responses, (*b*) patients' beliefs about the situations they encounter, and (*c*) their inferred ability to deal with their challenges. The subjective distress may take the form of vague feelings of terror, threat or impending disaster/catastrophe as seen in panic attacks or generalized anxiety disorder. Alternatively, subjective distress may involve specific thoughts and images, for instance, in the case of a patient suffering from a phobia of dogs who, during assessment, may report images of being bitten by a dog. Further, particular thoughts and images may also be recalled by phobic individuals, for example, agoraphobic patients may report nightmares of having a panic attack sometime in the future and that they may not be able to deal with it.

From the non-behavioral perspective, anxiety is understood, either in terms of the stimulus situation which may give rise to anxiety, or as a trait or characteristic of the individual's personality. Freud, in his writings, differentiated between "objective" anxiety and "neurotic" anxiety by the presence or absence of an objectively threatening stimulus. Objective anxiety was considered by him as the response to a realistic threat (an oncoming vehicle in the wrong lane, the sound of footsteps in a dark alley), whereas neurotic anxiety was taken to be an irrational response to an internal conflict which had no objective or realistic basis (fear of aggressive impulses). Similarly, a differentiation is made between fear and anxiety, with fear being regarded as a response to an identifiable threat (such as closed spaces, darkness or heights), and anxiety regarded as a response to a threat which cannot be easily delineated (such as interpersonal anxiety experienced during social encounters).

However, experts believe that there cannot be reliable differences between subjective feelings, physiological/somatic arousal and motor behaviors. They are of the view that adequate assessment and analysis would reveal that there almost always exists a specific, threatening stimulus which is predominantly cognitive in nature and is experienced by the patient at times as being laughed at/or losing control over self, thereby making anxiety as a construct vague and diffused.

Manifestation of anxiety

As mentioned earlier, anxiety manifests itself differently in different persons. In some, it has an effect on the cardiovascular system (palpitations, sweating), in others on the gastrointestinal system (nausea, vomiting, diarrhea), or the genito-urinary system (increased urination frequency). In addition to these manifestations, anxiety may be seen in muscle tension or spasms, headache or a wry neck. Anxiety is a chronic feeling of discomfort due to repeated stimuli that activate the ergotropic, autonomic nervous system and create an excessive discharge in the visceral and motor systems. Some of the mental and bodily signs and symptoms that accompany anxiety are presented in Box 1.1.

Box 1.1: Commonly reported bodily signs and symptoms in anxiety

Respiratory system	*Alimentary and excretory system*
Breathlessness	Lump in throat
Shortness of breath	Dryness of mouth
Sighing	"Butterflies" in stomach
Pressure on chest	Passing of wind
Choking sensation	Diarrhea—Enhanced urinary function, hesitancy, urgency
Skeletal-muscular system	*Others*
Shaking/trembling	Disturbed sleep patterns
Tension headaches	Nightmares
"Wobbly legs"	Restlessness and pacing
Stuttering/stammering	Pins and needles sensation
Rapid speech	Numbing sensation
Muscle cramps	Difficulty in thinking
	Bodily pains and tiredness

Anxiety and stress

Although the terms "anxiety" and "stress" are often used synonymously, either of these can cause the other. The term "stress" may also be used with two meanings, viz., (*a*) the stimuli that trigger the chronic state of anxiety and (*b*) the inability of the individual to cope with an external or internal event. Both these lead to exaggerated and prolonged anxiety, causing high levels of autonomic responses. While the former is called the stressor, the latter is called stress. It may be emphasized here that every stress does not necessarily lead to anxiety. An event being stressful depends on (*a*) its nature (*b*) the resources available to the individual to deal with it and (*c*) the coping mechanisms used by the individual. Thus, depending on any of these three aspects, stress may be severe, leading to intense anxiety.

conflict

Conflict is considered an essential part of anxiety. It may arise due to (*a*) external events, called "inter-personal" and (*b*) internal events, called "intra-psychic". Whenever conflict arises it causes anxiety which may manifest itself in the physical, psychical and behavioral areas. Distress due to the conflict may be observed at the (*a*) neuro-endocrine level (*b*) motor-visceral level (*c*) level of conscious awareness or (*d*) in all three simultaneously.

Explicitly stated, when a person complains of anxiety, the associated symptoms and signs may manifest themselves in any or all of physiological, psychological and behavioral areas. In physiological manifestations of anxiety, the person may experience palpitations, dizziness/feeling faint, muscle tension, wobbly legs, sweaty palms, etc. In the psychological realm, it may affect the person's thoughts and perception resulting in inaccurate perception of danger, underestimation of his/her ability to cope, endless worry of things that can go wrong, or underestimation of the help available to him. In addition, psychological manifestation of anxiety may take the form of emotional disturbances which can be observed in the person being nervous, edgy, panicky or irritable. Anxiety also brings about a change in the person which can be seen in his avoiding or walking out of situations that arouse anxiety.

Generally, a person with anxiety is conscious of a disagreeable feeling that has two components: (*a*) the awareness of the physiological sensations such as palpitations, sweating and tightness in the chest and (*b*) the realization of being disproportionately nervous or frightened and its irrationality. Another fear is related to his anxiety about whether others perceive him in a bad light because of his irrational behavior.

Severe anxiety, as mentioned earlier, might also lead to distortion in perception of time, space and person, as well as in the meaning attached to events. Such distortions may interfere with the cognitive and behavioral aspects of the person in such a way as to lower his efficiency in learning, attention, concentration, retention and memory. They may also decrease his ability to relate and associate one event with another. Because of these distortions, such a person tends to select only certain items in the environment to which to respond, overlooking other important aspects that are necessary in order to understand a situation in the right perspective. This selective perception and thinking affects not only the inclusion of inappropriate events, but also the exclusion of regular events, people and things, resulting in incorrect understanding of the meaning of words and actions of others.

While anxiety may be negative and might cause discomfort, it may also be positive and act as an alerting signal. It warns the person of an impending threat (external or internal), and causes pain and helplessness that may take the form of possible self-punishment, or separation from loved ones, threat to one's success or status, or may be even a threat to one's unity, balance and wholeness. On being thus alerted by anxiety, the individual is moved to take steps necessary to prevent the danger/threat. Where such prevention is not possible, efforts are focused on lessening the impact of the threat. The steps taken by the individual towards reduction or prevention of the impact of threat include many strategies and defense mechanisms, and the moment the threat passes and balance is restored, the defenses are given up until a similar threatening episode occurs. Such strategies (neurotic defenses) help the individual to overcome anxiety and, in the process, get reinforced as they reduce anxiety and restore balance. In due course of time, these defense strategies become a part of the person's behavior and are used for handling unpleasant and threatening situations that may be encountered from time to time. This pattern tends to replace the existing, normal coping strategies and behaviors, and when a difficult or unpleasant situation arises, neurotic behavior rises to the fore. Thus, anxiety becomes an extremely negative condition leading to the onset of many neurotic disorders. When anxiety is the most pronounced feature of these conditions, different types of anxiety disorders are encountered as shown in Box 1.2.

Box 1.2: Major anxiety disorders with their core symptomatology

Anxiety disorders	Core symptoms
Agoraphobia	Extreme anxiety and fear characterized by avoidance of places or situations in which escape may be difficult or help not available.
Specific phobia	Extreme and uncontrollable fear of a specific object or situation (animals, blood, thunder, being in public places etc.).
Social phobia	Extreme and uncontrollable anxiety regarding fear of scrutiny, humiliation and embarrassment in social settings, such as eating out in restaurants or making presentations, which are avoided by the individual.
Obsessive-compulsive disorder	Intrusive, senseless thoughts or images (wanting to kill someone, thinking that the child will get hurt), accompanied by stereotyped ritualistic behaviors (washing hands, foot-tapping or mental counting). However much the individual tries to stop these thoughts and actions, they return with greater force, causing further anxiety.
Post-traumatic stress disorder	Extreme anxiety experienced by the patient when s/he re-experiences a traumatic event accompanied by avoidance of the stimuli associated with trauma.
Acute stress disorder	Symptoms are almost similar to those obtained in the post-traumatic stress disorder, occurring within four weeks following an extremely traumatic event and causing severe anxiety.
Anxiety due to a general medical condition	Prominent symptoms of anxiety due to physiological consequences of a general medical condition.

(Box 1.2 continued)

| Substance-induced anxiety disorder | Prominent symptoms of anxiety due to physiological consequences of drug abuse, toxins or medications, or due to withdrawal of the drugs (withdrawal symptoms). |
| Anxiety disorder Not Otherwise Specified (NOS) | Symptoms of anxiety for which there is inadequate or contradictory information. |

Anxiety can also be one of the main symptoms reported by a person suffering from disorders such as depression, schizophrenia or disorders caused by organic factors. Hence, it is necessary to differentiate anxiety disorders from all other disorders where anxiety is equally severe so as to arrive at the correct diagnosis.

Differential Diagnosis of Anxiety Disorders

Panic disorder

The diagnosis for a patient with panic disorder requires that the disorder be clearly differentiated from malingering, hypochondriasis, depersonalization disorder, social and specific phobias, post-traumatic stress disorder, depressive disorders and schizophrenia. By definition, panic disorder is characterized by recurrent, spontaneous, uncued, "out of the blue" panic attacks. These attacks can be of three types—unexpected, situationally bound, and situationally predisposed. The presence of recurrent and unexpected panic attacks either initially or at a later stage in the course of the disorder is required for an adequate diagnosis of panic disorder. However, panic attacks that occur in the context of other anxiety disorders are situationally bound or predisposed (for example, in social phobia they are cued by social situations, in specific phobias by an object or situation, in obsessive-compulsive disorder by the exposure to the object of obsession, and in post-traumatic stress disorder, to recalling the stressor.

When criteria are met for both panic disorder and another anxiety or mood disorder, both should be diagnosed. However, when unexpected panic attacks occur in the context of another disorder (as in the case of a major depressive disorder or generalized anxiety disorder) but are not accompanied by other episodes of panic attacks and related somatic or cognitive symptoms within a month of the first such episode, then the additional diagnosis of panic disorder is not made. Furthermore, panic disorder is not diagnosed if the panic attacks are judged to be a physiological effect of a general medical condition (hyperthyroidism, multiple sclerosis, epilepsy, pulmonary diseases, cardiac conditions etc.). Appropriate medical examination needs to be carried out to determine the etiological role of such diseases in causing panic disorder. Diagnosis of panic disorder is also not made if panic attacks are judged to be the result of a substance intake (abuse of drug, effect of medication), in which case a substance-induced anxiety disorder is diagnosed. Intoxication due to stimulants (cocaine, caffeine, amphetamines) or withdrawal from depressants (alcohol or barbiturates) can also precipitate a panic attack, but if the attacks persist long after the effects of intoxication or cessation of withdrawal symptoms, a diagnosis of panic disorder should be considered.

Specific phobias

Specific phobias differ from other anxiety disorders in levels of intermittent anxiety. Typically, patients with specific phobias do not present pervasive anxiety but show anxiety only in limited cases of specific, circumscribed objects or situations. In addition, in specific phobias of situational types, there are no unexpected panic attacks as long as the patient avoids the anxiety-arousing situation. Differentiation between a specific phobia and panic disorder with agoraphobia may be particularly difficult because both these disorders include panic attacks and avoidance of similar types of situations, such as flying, drinking, travelling in public transport and being in enclosed places. However, three important features distinguish agoraphobia from anxiety disorder: in agoraphobia (*a*) multiple situations may spark off panic attacks (*b*) these panic attacks occur unexpectedly, with an intensity that frightens the patient and (c) the patient starts avoiding situations that trigger the panic attacks.

Some patients may manifest symptoms that fall between agoraphobia and specific phobias. These need to be thoroughly assessed and a proper clinical judgment made for an appropriate diagnosis. For example, an individual who had not previously feared or avoided elevators suddenly experiences a panic attack in an elevator, which frightens him to such an extent that he dreads going to work because he has to take the elevator to his office. If such panic attacks subsequently occur only in elevators and not in any other situations, then a diagnosis of specific phobia may be appropriate. However, if the individual experiences unexpected panic attacks in other situations also and begins to avoid those because of fear of a panic attack, then a diagnosis of panic disorder with agoraphobia should be made. Specific and social phobias are differentiated on the basis of the focus of fear. Avoidance of eating in a restaurant may be based on concerns about being negatively evaluated by others (social phobia) or about choking in a closed room (specific phobia). In contrast to what is obtained in a specific phobia, avoidance in post-traumatic disorder follows life-threatening stressors and is accompanied by intense features as re-experiencing the trauma and the restricted affect. Avoidance in obsessive-compulsive disorder is, on the other hand, associated with the content of obsession (dirt, contamination).

Differentiation between hypochondriasis and specific phobias of the illness type is made on the grounds that, in case of the former, the patient fears having the disease whereas in the latter there is fear of contracting the disease. An individual with schizophrenia or any psychotic disorder may avoid certain activities in response to delusions, but there is no recognition of these activities unlike in specific phobia cases where the fear is excessive, irrational or unreasonable.

Social phobia

As has been pointed out earlier, in social phobias a person avoids public places due to the fear of evaluation of his actions by others, even though in reality no such evaluation occurs. Thus, anxiety here is directly related to others and to social situations with the resultant behavior being that of avoiding all types of social situations.

In schizoid personality disorder, social situations are avoided because of a lack of interest in relating to other individuals. In contrast, social phobia patients have a capacity for and are interested in social relationships with familiar people. Performance anxiety, stage fright, and shyness in social situations with unfamiliar people are common and should not be diagnosed as social phobia unless the anxiety or avoidance leads to significant impairment and marked distress. The avoidance of social situations is one of the symptoms of depression. However, a thorough assessment would elicit the typical constellation of depressive symptoms on the basis of which a diagnosis of depression can be made.

Obsessive-compulsive disorder

An individual with obsessive-compulsive disorder may have recurrent thoughts, ideas or images which are generally obnoxious, and so, are resisted. However, the more the person resists these thoughts, the greater is the intensity with which they reappear. The anxiety here is thus directly related to recurrent, unpleasant and obnoxious thoughts, and the person is helpless in being unable to prevent these from occurring. Attempts to deal with these are through certain repetitive acts and purposeful behaviors (washing hands, counting steps) which are recognized as irrational and potentially embarrassing. In compulsions, the person is faced with an irresistible desire to do something repetitively although he knows that it is unwanted, silly, irrational and irrelevant. The more he resists, the greater is the intensity of his compulsion. Compulsive responses may be central as well as peripheral. Such obsessions and repetitions of an idea together with the increasing intensity of the resisted thoughts are present in anxiety.

Obsessive-compulsive disorder is to be distinguished from anxiety disorder due to a general medical condition. A diagnosis of the latter is made when obsessions and compulsions are due to the direct physiological consequences of a general medical condition (Tourette's disorder, temporal lobe epilepsy and postencephalitic complication).

Recurrent intrusive thoughts, impulses, image or behaviors may occur in the context of many other mental disorders. The diagnosis of obsessive-compulsive disorder is not made if these thoughts and compulsions are exclusive to another disorder (preoccupation with bodily appearance as in body dystrophic disorder, hair pulling in trichotillomania, kleptomania, and so on).

If the obsessive, intrusive thoughts are related to the fear of having a serious disease then a diagnosis of hypochondraisis should be made. However, if concerns of having an illness are accompanied by rituals such as excessive repetitive or checking behavior, or if the worries are concerned with the fear that others around will acquire the disease, then an additional diagnosis of obsessive-compulsive disorder may be warranted.

The absence of the typical symptoms of schizophrenia combined with the less bizarre nature of the disorder help in differentiating obsessive personality disorder from schizophrenia. Further, the ruminative, delusional thoughts that occur in schizophrenia are distinguished from obsessions and thoughts by the fact that they are not ego-dystonic. In instances where a patient manifests symptoms of obsessive-compulsive disorder and schizophrenia, a diagnosis of both may be made.

Post-traumatic stress disorder

Another disorder that needs to be differentially diagnosed from anxiety disorders is post-traumatic stress disorder (PTSD). In this the person, on recall of an event either in dreams or flashbacks (that involved actual or threatened death), experiences severe anxiety. This disorder is distinguished from acute stress disorder on the basis of the fact that in the latter, the symptoms occur within four weeks of the traumatic event and are resolved within those four weeks. If the symptoms persist for more than a month and meet the criteria for post-traumatic stress disorder, then this should be diagnosed. In obsessive-compulsive disorder, there are recurrent intrusive thoughts, and not flashbacks or appearances in dreams, as in PTSD. Furthermore, these are experienced as inappropriate by obsessive-compulsive disorder patients and are not related to an experienced, traumatic event.

Anxiety due to a general medical condition

Since patients suffering from anxiety disorders manifest many physical and psychological symptoms, it is imperative to rule out organic factors that could have initiated, exacerbated or maintained the symptoms. A detailed case history will be able to provide the needed information to rule out organicity. If any doubts remain, a second medical opinion regarding the person's physical condition may be sought from the physician who has treated the patient. Physical impairment often complicates overt anxiety problems. It should be kept in mind, however, that as soon as the organic factor is identified and the patient takes the prescribed medicine, the accompanying anxiety recedes along with a disappearance or reduction in the intensity of the physical discomfort. Common medical conditions that lead to symptoms of anxiety include hyperthyroidism, Cushing's syndrome, hypoglycemia, temporal lobe epilepsy, and so on. Laboratory tests and a physical examination may be helpful in arriving at a diagnosis. If panic attacks are judged as the direct physiological consequence of a general medical condition, a diagnosis of anxiety disorder due to a general medical condition should be made.

Substance-induced anxiety disorder

Anxiety symptoms commonly occur both in substance intoxication and substance withdrawal. Under conditions where the anxiety symptoms are judged to be more than those usually associated with intoxication or withdrawal syndrome, a diagnosis of substance-induced anxiety disorder is to be made instead of substance intoxication or substance withdrawal. This diagnosis is made, particularly when anxiety symptoms are sufficiently severe as to warrant independent clinical attention. In other situations, if panic attacks continue outside of substance abuse ·(long after the effects of intoxication or withdrawal have ended), are recurring and unexpected, and are situation bound and situationally predisposed, a diagnosis of panic disorder will be made.

Generalized anxiety disorders

It is important to distinguish Generalized Anxiety Disorders from anxiety disorder due to a general medical condition. A diagnosis of the latter is made if the symptoms of anxiety are due to the direct physiological effect of a general medical condition such as cardiovascular disease, pulmonary disease, neurological disease etc. Similarly, substance-induced anxiety disorder is distinguished from generalized anxiety disorder by the fact that a substance is judged to be etiologically related to the anxiety disorder. Generalized anxiety is a common, associated feature of mood disorder and psychotic disorders. It is not diagnosed separately if it occurs exclusively during the course of these conditions. Likewise, generalized anxiety disorder is not diagnosed if the anxiety occurs exclusively during the course of the post-traumatic disorder.

Thus, anxiety disorders manifest in a variety of symptoms and ways, differentially in different persons and situations and with varying intensity. While anxiety is experienced by almost every person, in some it works as a positive force driving them towards bettering their own performance, while in others, it is like any normal day-to-day emotion and is handled routinely. For yet others, anxiety works as a negative force affecting adversely their efficiency, performance and daily routine. Although anxiety reduces performance levels, its very presence brings about a state of balance in a person. This, in turn, reinforces it as and when any stressful event takes place. Thus, anxiety becomes a routine, regular pattern of behavior used by the person to restore his mental balance. When anxiety becomes overwhelming and incapacitates the individual, it leads to the development of anxiety disorders.

2
Etiology of Anxiety Disorders

Anxiety Disorders—Theoretical Perspectives

Different theories of personality attempt to explain the psycho-pathology and symptomatology of psychiatric disorders from varying perspectives. No one theory can explain human behavior satisfactorily or adequately account for the many disorders encountered in clinical practice. Theories which explain psycho-pathology and the underlying psychodynamics also provide treatment techniques to handle these problems. This chapter explains, with the help of a few major theories, the psychopathologies encountered in psychiatric settings.

Psychoanalytical theory

Psychoanalytical theory is one of the most frequently used theories explaining psychiatric disorders. Sigmund Freud's theory of anxiety emphasized biological genesis in the sexual instinct, thus attributing pathological anxiety to disturbances in sexual functions. The theory also made a distinction between the etiological factors that produced anxiety, neurasthenia, hypochondriasis and anxiety disorders, and those that caused hysteria and somatoform disorder.

In Freud's theory, dreams occupy a central position in both the diagnosis and the treatment of psychiatric disorders. The analysis of dreams reveals materials that have been repressed or excluded from the consciousness of the patient by the defensive activities of the ego. These repressed materials, by manifesting themselves in dreams, serve to discharge latent impulses. Thus, they protect the person from excessive anxiety and pain.

Another important concept is that of the "unconscious", which contains the repressed ideas, desires, and negative experiences that are inaccessible to the "conscious" realm of the individual. The unconscious also makes use of primitive mental operations such as displacement. This helps in rapidly discharging the mental energy which is attached to these mental ideas. Freud pointed out that repression of childhood memories occurs if energy is withdrawn from the verbal expression of these materials.

According to psychoanalytical theory, while the mental energy associated with unconscious ideas seeks discharge through thought or motor activities, under certain conditions its direction is reversed. Thus, childhood impressions in their original form appear in dreams or as hallucinations in psychiatric patients. One of the principal functions of the ego is to maintain a relationship with the external world by sensing, testing, and adapting to reality. In the early stages of development, these defensive measures emerge due to the ego's struggle to mediate between the pressures of id and the requirements of outside reality. However, as the individual grows, many of these develop into typical patterns of behavior resulting in neurotic tendencies because of alterations in the normal, defensive functioning of the ego.

Another explanation for psychopathology in psychoanalytical theory is the concept of superego, which comes into being with the resolution of the Oedipus complex. Freud was of the view that in real anxiety, a threat emanates from known dangers outside of the individual, while in neurotic anxiety the threat is perceived from an unknown danger that may not necessarily be external. The individual concerned attempts to ward off these threats by the use of defense mechanisms which, according to Freud, include reaction formation, regression, repression, sublimation, undoing, and displacement. These responses of the ego tend, at times, to become established patterns of behavior rather than remaining isolated instances. Being unsuited to the general, day-to-day demands of living, the behavior turns out to be maladaptive.

While discussing the stages of psychosexual development, Freud pointed out that over-gratification or deprivation of oral needs can result in libidinal fixation that contributes to pathological traits, such as excessive optimism, narcissism, pessimism (often seen in depressive states), and a high degree of dependency, envy, and jealousy.

Of the different stages of psychosexual development, the anal period is essentially a period of striving for independence, and separation from the dependence and control of the parents. Maladaptive behaviors arise from anal eroticism and the defenses against it. Orderliness, obstinacy, stubbornness, willfulness, frugality, and parsimony are features of anal characters and are derived from a fixation on the anal stage. When defenses against anal traits are less effective, the person reveals heightened ambivalence, lack of tidiness, messiness, defiance, rage, and sadomasochistic tendencies. These characteristics and defenses are most typically seen in obsessive-compulsive disorders.

Important distortions of the phallic stage arise from the patterns of identification developing out of the resolution of oedipal complex. The derivation of the pathological traits from the phallic oedipal involvement is so complex and subject to such a variety of modifications, that it encompasses nearly the whole body of neurotic disorders.

The latency stage is a period of relative quiescence or inactivity of sexual desire from the age of 5–6 years to 11–13 years. Problems in the latency period can arise either due to lack of development of inner controls, or an excess of inner controls. An excess of inner control can lead to premature closure of psychosexual development and the precocious elaboration of obsessive character traits.

In the genital stage, pathological deviations occur due to the failure to achieve successful resolution of this stage of development which are, in a sense, a partial reopening, reworking and reinterpreting of all earlier aspects of development. If these remained unresolved in previous phases, they produce pathological defects in the emerging adult, for example defects from a failure to resolve adolescent issues (called identity diffusion by *Erickson*, 1980).

During the course of development of an individual, many factors contribute to the malfunctioning and malformation of the psychic self. Need deprivation in the first few months of life, for example, may impair ego development with devastating effects on its integrative capacities. At a still higher stage of development, an individual's failure to make necessary identifications, either because of over indulgence or excessive frustration, may interfere with the ego's ability to mediate between instinct and environment. The lack of integrative capacities of the ego may result in two kinds of psychopathology. In one, the person develops a high degree of suspicion that his needs will not be fulfilled, thereby manifesting fears and insecurities in the form of paranoid symptoms. In the second, the person becomes extremely withdrawn from a world that gives only pain (as in schizophrenia). When the ego lacks the capacity to balance between the instinct and the outside world, the manifestation of psychopathology is in the form of hostility and aggression. These may be turned towards the self or directed towards others. In case of the former, it may manifest in depression, suicidal ideation, suicidal attempts or self-punishment, and in the latter, it may take the form of an antisocial personality disorder, psychopathic personality or aggressive conduct disorder.

Another important explanation for the onset of neurotic disorders are the precipitating factors. These are external to the individual and their intensity and unpleasantness may disturb his mental and emotional balance, forcing him to react in a way which involves conflict between warded off impulses and warding off forces. The resulting psychopathology takes the form of neurotic disorders. The psychoanalytical explanation of these disorders involves basically a struggle between the warding off of one's undesirable impulses (which threaten to cause shame and guilt) and those forces from the environment which constantly obstruct need gratification.

Freud was of the view that an increase in sexual tension leads to a corresponding increase in the mental representation of the sexual instinct, together with a variety of associated ideas and emotions. Further interference with the adequate discharge of the psychic component of sexual tension gives rise to anxiety. In hysteria and obsessive-compulsive disorder, there is interference in the normal libidinal functioning due to psychic conflict or repression. One of the theories of anxiety is of toxic/physiological origin which says that dammed up and undischarged libido is forced to seek physical discharge in the form of an anxiety symptom. The second theory is related to the patients' sexual malfunctioning and says that the cause of anxiety lies in a greater and specifically more psychological level viz., in the repression of libidinal urges that are typically thought of as derived from unconscious, infantile memories.

As Freud replaced the topographical model of the mind with the structural model, anxiety was considered in terms of the dangers to the ego rather than due to repression. Accordingly, neurotic symptoms such as phobias were seen as indicative of a partial defect in the defensive function of the ego, resulting in a distortion of its relationship with certain aspects of the outside world. From this point of view of Freud, in these anxiety states, the ego is no longer passive, helpless or vulnerable against the demands of the id as well as the outside world. In fact, it is capable of defending itself against all such demands through reaction formation, isolation and undoing. Thus, obsessive-compulsive disorder comes about due to the ego's defense mechanisms of undoing and isolation wherein there is separation of affect (emotions) from ideas or behaviors or by regression to the anal sadistic stage or turning the impulses against self. The depressive disorder, on the other hand, involves reaction to loss or to failure such as the death of a loved object or disappointment with a loved one. There may also be a discrepancy between the values maintained by the superego and the behavior of the individual, evoking punishment in the form of guilt and leading to low self-esteem in depressives.

Each form of neurotic disorder has its characteristic secondary gains. In anxiety disorder there is regression to childhood a period where one was still protected. In dissociative and conversion disorders there is the material gain of attention from others because of dramatic acting out. In compulsive disorders, there is narcissistic gain through pride and illness and in somatoform disorders, psychic conflicts are denied by projecting them onto the physical sphere.

The etiological explanation of disorders in psychoanalytical theory led to the treatment method of psychoanalysis in which free association and dream analysis techniques are used to elicit materials repressed in the unconscious. Resistance is commonly encountered while retrieving these materials and the therapist can infer this by the patient's pauses in the interview or in his coming late for appointments or by slips of the tongue during conversations. Other indicators of resistance include stammering, remaining silent, fidgeting with some part of the clothing or asking irrelevant questions. Understanding this resistance, helps the therapist use techniques such as dream interpretation, clarification, and insight development. Transference may also be used, where the patient projects his past, repressed feelings and emotions onto the therapist. This reduces resistance and helps the patient move forward easily in his therapeutic process. In the course of analysis, the patient goes through two processes viz., remembering and reliving, both of which constitute the dynamic part of the psychoanalytic treatment procedure. This not only reduces the intensity of the event but also helps the patient learn to deal with such events more adequately.

In recent years, considerable modifications have been effected in the methods and techniques of classical psychoanalysis, for example, the inclusion of sociocultural components in both diagnosis and treatment. Psychoanalysts associated with these modifications include Alfred Adler, Eric Fromm, Karen Horney, Harry Stack Sullivan and Otto Rank, all of whom are referred to as Neo-Freudians.

According to Adlerian theory, a neurotic disposition stems from childhood experiences characterized by overprotection, neglect or confusion, or an alternating mixture of these. Such experiences create a negative image of helplessness in the growing child and convince him that he does not posses the ability to master or cope with the varied demands of life. This distorted image of the helpless self is supplemented by the individual's perception of the social environment as being hostile, punitive, depriving, and frustrating. Negative early experiences provide misleading cues to the child and prevent him from having a cognitive map suited to the tasks of social life. This, in turn, discourages him from putting in any effort towards mastery and achievement, leaving him fearful and de-motivated. Thus, instead of experiencing the pleasures of a trusting and loving relationship, the child becomes distrustful and manipulative. He develops a neurotic striving for superiority to compensate for exaggerated feelings of anxiety and inferiority, his main objective being self-protection and self-centeredness. He uses non-cooperation for achieving his goals, solving problems from a self-centered rather than task-centered point of view. This life goal is shaped negatively with fears and anxiety, with subjectivity disturbing his awareness of objective reality—all of which threatens his self-image. Furthermore, since he is afraid of facing new, corrective experiences and avoids the human contact that could help him clarify many distortions, his faulty assumptions remain at large and his neurotic behavior remains unchanged.

The treatment technique of the Adlerian approach consists of psychotherapy. This attempts to mobilize the patient's creative resources and helps him achieve cognitive re-organization. The result is a less rigid and more accurate appraisal of reality, better relationships with others, and fulfillment of creative potential. Adler believed that this process of re-education should start from childhood and advocated Child Guidance Clinics so that children could experience love, care and nurturance in a positive manner and not have to suffer from insecurity and negative self image.

Eric Fromm, another psychoanalyst who had included socio-cultural factors in his explanation of disorders, considered man's behavior as being motivated by his biological requirements. According to him, human motivation and behavior were culturally determined, with society generating new needs and problems. These, when superimposed on man's instinctual needs, become as imperative as the demands of hunger, thirst, and sex. He explained neurotic disorders, including masochism, sadism, conformity, automation and neurosis as man's attempts to escape from the basic dichotomy in human existence. Based on his theorization, Fromm put forward five types of personality, each of which explained typical behavior patterns in individuals. These are as follows:

> *Receptive character*—in which the individual keeps receiving but never gives or shares with others.
> *Exploitative character*—in which the individual exploits others for his own good.
> *Hoarding character*—in which the individual tries to save the maximum, even to the extent of hoarding, so that his future is secure.
> *Marketing character*—in which the individual manipulates others to achieve his ends.
> *Productive character*—in which the individual contributes positively.

Karen Horney, who parted company with Freud, presented a redefinition of neurosis in which attention was shifted from specific symptoms to total personality disturbances. Horney conceptualized neurosis as a disturbance in total personality with its source in:

a) Distorted parent–child relationship, subsequently self perpetuating.
b) Distortions in relationships with others and self, stemming from emotional conflicts, anxiety, and unconscious, intrapsychic efforts to avoid the disintegrative efforts of these conflicts.
c) Discrepancies between potential and actual achievement.

Horney was one of the first psychoanalysts to stress the importance of cultural influences. In putting forward the psychodynamics of the neurotic process, Karen Horney said early childhood experiences played a crucial role in the genesis of a neurosis. An

infant subjected to a variety of neurotically determined parental
attitudes (excessive parental expectations, over-strictness, smoth-
ering love or rejection), feels uncomfortable and develops a distorted personality. To counteract parental attitudes, he tends to
develop those reactions or traits that best ensure feelings of security and safety. Despite the biological dependency universal all
infants, they react to their parents in different ways, classified by
Horney into three groups:

a) Moving towards people by accepting love, closeness and
   dependency on the mothering one, and others associated
   with the same.
b) Moving away from people into solitude, privacy and self
   containment.
c) Moving against people through friction, self-assertion and
   protest.

The child exposed to rejecting parental attitudes reacts with vague
feelings of loneliness, helplessness and fear of a potentially hostile world. Such a reaction is termed as "basic anxiety" by Horney
who further opines that a child, in order to avoid this anxiety,
develops certain neurotic trends or drives such as compulsive
aggression, submission or detachment. One of these attitudes
usually predominates, while the others are repressed but continue to exert a dynamic force. Thus, anxiety is the mainspring
from where such attitudes develop and gain pervasiveness. In line
with her theoretical propositions, Horney suggested three possible
solutions: (a) self-effacement (b) expansiveness and (c) resignation.
In addition, she suggested auxiliary solutions such as "externaliza-
tion" of inner processes or feelings as occurring outside of the self,
"compartmentalization" that is, experiencing the self as consisting
of unconnected parts, and "alienation" from self as both a defensive
measure and a neurotic process.

Childhood is considered the most important period in the
development of a neurosis. The emphasis in this therapy is on
the present and its main goal is to make the unconscious, conscious. Gross movement during analysis may take any of three
forms, namely disillusionment, reorientation, and mobilization

of constructive forces. Treatment techniques include the psycho-analytic techniques mentioned earlier.

Instead of postulating a maternal instinct to explain the domineering interest of the mother in her child, H.S. Sullivan emphasized that the tension of the infant's need stimulates anxiety in the mother which is manifested as the care, attention and tenderness that the infant requires. Sullivan maintained that man is simply "more human than otherwise", implying that in the performance of his diverse activities, man is closer to the human mode of functioning than to that of animals. The presence of anxiety is considered central to human development. The varying amounts of anxiety in an individual determine his variable state of euphoria. Sullivan views anxiety as a creative force as well as an inevitable accompaniment to human growth. All humans have major goals which he termed as end state. The first of these is to fulfil the biological needs of the organism (food, air, sex etc.) and is called the need for survival. The second goal relates to man as an uncultured being and involves those needs that go beyond the purely physiological ones and is called the need for security. He also distinguished three different modes of experiencing and termed them parataxic, prototaxic and syntaxic.

Sullivan viewed personality development as the process of learning to handle anxiety using adaptive maneuvers and defensive techniques. His concept of anxiety is valuable in the psychological treatment of mental disorders, as the presence of anxiety facilitates identification of the patients' problems and highlights those elements of their personality which meet with the therapist's approval. According to Sullivan, unfortunate, past experiences lead people to develop views, attitudes, and beliefs about themselves that often differ widely from those of the expert. These distorted viewpoints forever trap them or compel them into incongruous and inappropriate situations, often with great harm to themselves or others.

Sullivan considered anxiety as both a positive and a negative force. In explaining mental disorders, he believed that certain tendencies were dissociated in a neurosis and dealt with by substitutive tendencies, for example, displacement and distraction.

In the obsessive-compulsive disorder, on the other hand, the insecurities of the individual are held in check by the substitutive device of magic and is controlled by ritual. In hysteria, the substitutive technique used is amnesia, in which clear recognition of issues is avoided and somatic substitutions become the major area of relating to others.

Sullivan considers psychiatry as the study of interpersonal processes and his concept of pathology is intimately tied to the self-system that develops as a result of the need to reduce anxiety. The focus of Sullivan's therapy is not only on anxiety but also on the entire gamut of interpersonal contexts in which it occurs. The therapy helps the patient to reconstruct his individual functioning in as balanced a manner as possible, and to strengthen his self-esteem, thus enabling him to effectively handle the contexts and relationships that provoke anxiety.

Otto Rank put forth the concept of birth trauma. Till the time of birth, the infant grows in the comfortable environment of an even temperature with all his needs automatically taken care of. At the time of birth, however, not only has he to come out of that comfortable cocoon but also has to travel a long, hazardous path. Finally, he is pushed out into a world in which he has to learn to breathe, swallow and ingest on his own and adjust to the heat and cold of the environment. The process of birth and the subsequent adjustments are all highly unpleasant and, in some cases, may be so traumatic as to cause severe anxiety called birth trauma. The anxiety experienced at the time of birth continues to be imbedded in the individual's life to such an extent that despite years of growth and development, it remains with the person and influences the various aspects of his life. The manner in which the person learns to handle it decides his personality traits. Thus, Otto Rank identified three types of personality—artistic or creative, neurotic and antisocial, and normal. In the treatment, which he called relationship therapy, Rank emphasized the relationship between patient and therapist. The treatment's goal is to help the patient accept his separateness and will. Thus, throughout therapy the patient is given the quiet assurance that he can be loved without feeling that he is being dominated.

Eric Erikson maintained that a person grows throughout life interacting continually with the environment and faces conflicts at all stages of development. The conflict, therefore, is seen as a continuing and inseparable process between early, primitive values and later, mature ones. With a good, functioning ego, a person is not neurotically suffering, crippled or wasting his energy. A normal person can veer off the normal course because of problems within himself, within his interpersonal relations or within the society to which he attempts to adapt. When these interpersonal relationships become negative, they cause anxiety. Although anxiety is natural to all human beings, in infancy the difference between anxiety and fear is not known. However, when these fears persist into adulthood, they turn into neurotic anxieties.

Erikson put forward five physical modes of reaction to negative interpersonal reactions, viz., passive and active, incorporation, retention, elimination and intrusion. These underlie five social modes, viz., getting, taking, holding, letting go and being on the make or making. These modes operate sequentially and relate to different zones of the body namely, oral-sensory, muscular-anal, and locomotor-genital. A mismatch between the mode and the zone may lead to a neurotic pattern of behavior in the individual.

Learning theories

Theorists of this school are of the view that all behaviors (including pathological behaviors) are learned and can hence be unlearned. Neurotic behaviors may be precipitated by diverse types of stress including:

failure to live upto one's own expectations and those of others, with subsequent feelings of inferiority and failure, unexpected desires and weak spots arising from early trauma, seemingly impossible choices or decisions, dissonant cognition, and frustrating life situations that rob meaning and hope from life.

The antecedents of maladaptive behavior have to be identified and dealt with. Starting with the classical conditioning theory of

Ivan Pavlov which demonstrated that a behavior could be changed by using reinforcement associated with a particular unconditional or natural stimulus (that elicited the desired response), came a series of behavior modification techniques based on the instrumental conditioning of Skinner and the modeling approaches of Dollard and Miller. The techniques, which were initially tried on animals, were tried on humans with success by many experts such as Watson who demonstrated instilling and removing fear (phobia) of animals in a child.

In their experiment to demonstrate that humans learn and unlearn normal and abnormal behaviors, Watson and Raynor (1920) demonstrated the development of phobia in 11-month old Albert. They first showed that Albert was not afraid of furry objects and that he had no fear of any furry animals etc. He was then given a rat to play with and as he neared it, they produced fear by making a loud noise and Albert withdrew from the rat. This instilling of fear continued until after sometime not only was Albert afraid of the rat, he had generalized the fear to other objects resembling it. This experimentally induced fear was released later by means of social imitation and direct reconditioning.

Today's behavioral approach and the underlying themas stem directly from developments that took place during the twentieth century in Russia and America. The efforts of Throndike and Watson helped to not only understand human behavior in terms of stimulus response, but were supplemented by countless lab experiments that contributed to several theories of learning. Originally derived from lab experiments, the assumptions of learning theories postulate that inasmuch as a disturbed behavior is "acquired", its evolution and treatment can also be understood within the framework of these theories.

All behaviors, whether maladaptive or adaptive, are consequences of the same basic principles of behavior acquisition and maintenance. It is either learned or unlearned and normal or abnormal in accordance with its social significance. All learning theories can be subsumed under two basic mechanisms: (a) Classical Respondent Conditioning derived from Pavlov's famous experiments and (b) Operant Instrumental Conditioning linked to Skinner's instrumental conditioning experiments. Basic to these theories are the Law of Effect (theory of Throndike) and the pleasure principle of Freud's psychoanalytical theory, both of which assign the highest priority to the immediate precipitants of behavior, de-emphasizing the role of remote, underlying, causal determinants important in the medical field. Regardless of the mechanisms of learning, the theory asserts, quite simply, that there are two types of abnormal behavior, viz., (*a*) behavioral deficits that result from a failure to learn and (*b*) maladaptive behavior that is a consequence of inappropriate learning.

Over the years, many behavior modification techniques have evolved, all of which share certain common features. Before starting therapy, for example, a thorough interview followed by behavioral analysis is essential. This helps in identifying the antecedent variables related to the disorder and the reinforcers that need to be used in the therapeutic sessions. Following this is self-monitoring and evaluation which help ascertain the diagnosis as well as decide the reinforcers to be used. These take the form of rewards or punishments and are used to either facilitate a desirable behavior or reduce or extinguish an undesirable one. Some of the commonly used behavior modification techniques include desensitization therapy, explosive therapy, token economy, time out method, shaping and modeling. Depending on the problem of a particular patient, a method is selected for use. Invariably, relaxation therapy is combined with behavior modification.

Learning theories take a totally different view from that of psychoanalytic theories where the etiology of normal and neurotic behaviors is concerned. For instance, these theories do not give much importance to the individual's past, but stress upon the "here and now" aspects of the person.

Existential theory

According to this theory humans exist first, and their unique choices define them. These very choices form and define their selfhood and essence of living. These theorists are of the view that man is nothing but what he makes of himself. How a person leads his life and how he acts depends on his willingness to see his situation clearly and on the manner in which he sees his relationship to the world and to others. The clarity with which one sees oneself free and purposeful, and the extent to which his acts are participatory decide his level of existence in the world. The human freedom is not a thing, a being instead; it is the being of humans. It refers to the freedom to choose and implies a finite number of alternatives since each choice precludes others. A person is limited by the facility of his body and the things around him, for example, self-deception is a choice, a commitment to a way of existence in which the person does not know or see what he denies. Another person may deny by choosing not to look. In addition, any denial of the truth of one's vision is a lapse of authenticity and thus falls into self-deception. Self-deception, thus, is the motivated refusal to attend explicitly to responses in a situation that one has organized and chosen to live in. Further, according to the existentialist theory, self-deception is the major motive force underlying psychopathology which, in turn, is dependent on the person being unwilling to (a) attend closely to his priorities and commitments (b) see the world and himself with awareness (c) spell out the way he operates in the world (d) spell out the way others around him operate, and (e) lay out his personal myth clearly by focussed, explicit attending.

These encounters are responsible for a person developing pathology as they are indicative of certain expected behaviors in daily life. The humanistic–existentialist theory believes that violation takes place because of self-deception leading, in turn, to the development of psychopathology. A violating situation is one in which the person's vision is disconfirmed, his integrity is jeopardized or not accepted, and in which his subjectivity is destroyed, forcing him to submit to another perspective.

According to the existential theory, the basis of all mental illness is the partial withdrawal of a person from the outer world to his inner world. Such withdrawal is considered to be one of egocentricity or autism and may be enriching or retarding. This theory believes that a person with a creative personality will be able to "be in the world" and also share his values with others, whereas the mentally ill person is one who is "alienated" from the others and has a distorted "being in the world". Thus, one may find egocentric preoccupation in the hysterical patient's distortions of bodily functions. On the other hand, the rigid, legalistic rituals of the obsessive person represent preoccupation with a high degree of perfection. Existentialism views anxiety as manifesting itself in numerous variations, for example, loss of physical functions, fear of death and helplessness. All these drive the person to erect defenses in the form of autistic withdrawal, egocentricity etc. In the therapeutic encounter, these anxieties are re-experienced by the patient. The relationship between therapist and patient continues until normal trust is established. The therapist diverts the attention of the patient from his hidden guilt and feelings of worthlessness and helps him to make use of her thwarted potentialities. The trust that develops in this relationship is highly therapeutic as its brings new found freedom to the patient and helps him to develop his potentialities in a positive direction.

Family systems theory

In the past few decades, a major conceptual reorientation has occured in several sectors of the scientific community, with the focus increasingly on the family of the patient who is undergoing treatment. Cybernetics, systems theory, communication theory, objects relations' theory, social role theory, ethnology and ecology have all contributed to a better understanding of the family dynamic processes and their effect at conscious and unconscious levels in childhood psychopathology. In quite a few cases, observing their children growing activates unresolved childhood conflicts in the parents. This affects the communication style between a patient and his parents and may manifest as scapegoating, double bind or schizophrenogenic type communication. It has also been demonstrated that the type and extent of psychopathology in an individual can be inferred from the frequently observed patterns of identification and projection between parents and their children. Here, parental projection of self or part of self to the child results in them dealing with it as though it was a part of them.

The family is a self-regulating, open system with a unique history and structure that constantly evolves because of the dynamic interaction between its subsystems. Individuals interacting in this share a complementarity of needs. Family development, life-cycle, homeostasis, identity, values, goals, congruence, symmetry, myths, rules, roles, structure, double bind, pseudocommunity etc, stem from the cultural background of the family. Research studies focussing on family dynamics and relation to pathological behaviors contribute greatly to the understanding of different mental disorders as well as set the stage for the use of a wide range of psychiatric interventions.

Life span theories

Developmental theories state that in the absence of unusual interferences an individual matures in orderly predictable ways. These can be codified in a variety of interrelated psychosociobiological sequential systems. Such a developmental framework of reference is commonly obtained in child psychiatry. It is not only essential to understand how age-appropriate behaviors are important, but also how the child reacts to different types of frustrations, injury, illness, separation, death etc. These reactions have considerable implications in adulthood or if the child develops psychological disorders. It is important to appreciate the wide range of normal variation within interrelated developmental sequences as these lay a vital foundation and are of central significance in the individual's later development. The personality of the patient must be viewed in the perspective of the interrelationship between his past, present and future and the focus must be on questions of regression–progression and transience–permanence rather than on state assessment.

While many theories have been advanced to explain pathological states such as neurosis, psychosis and somatoform disorders, each of these focus upon a particular concept or a construct and develops a technique of treatment in line with that theorization. All the theories described deal with anxiety and, since each theory looks at it from a different perspective, various treatment methods and techniques have been proposed. While it is neither possible nor adequate to consider the past and take a deterministic approach toward explaining behavior, any explanation of normal or abnormal behavior will be inadequate and inappropriate if the past is not considered. No single theory can account for all types of behavioral and mental disorders and the person in distress needs to be understood and handled keeping in mind his unique qualities, assets and potentials. It may, perhaps, be more appropriate to combine the theoretical positions as well as the dynamic concepts to understand, in totality, an individual's behavior. A combination of psychoanalytical theory, the neo-Freudian approach, the learning theorists' explanation of behavior and the existential viewpoints could be used to explain each case of mental disorder. Perhaps this is one of the reasons why, in the present day, emphasis is placed on an eclectic approach to diagnosis and treatment, rather than on any single theory.

Etiology of Anxiety Disorders

Every person experiences anxiety as part of day-to-day living, some more and some less than others, under different circumstances. Since, anxiety may well hinder the smooth and efficient functioning of individuals, the question arises as to why, when and under what conditions anxiety becomes a negative drive or a pathological condition requiring psychiatric or psychological intervention. There appears to be no single answer to these questions, as anxiety can arise due to multiple causes, some known and some unknown.

When anxiety is overwhelming and affects a person's normal functioning, it may need to be treated either by medicine or by some other means. Such anxiety may be one of the symptoms of a number of psychiatric disorders. Anxiety disorders, in particular, have as their central feature severe anxiety, which is highly distressing to the person. To understand and treat the patient successfully, it is important to identify the causes of this anxiety. Different schools of psychology have explained and identified different sources of anxiety, and these theories include the psychoanalytical, learning, biological and sociological theories briefly presented in the following section.

Psychoanalytical explanation for anxiety disorders

The etiology advanced for anxiety disorders by the psychoanalytical school is considered to be a relatively comprehensive one, as it takes into consideration repressed, unconscious material to explain the patient's behavior. Anxiety results due to the conflict between repressed, instinctual drives which try to enter into the conscious and the attempts of the ego and superego to prevent them. It is also a response to the danger or threat that an individual experiences due to inadequately repressed impulses or conflicts. Sigmund Freud, in 1926, proposed that dangerous and unacceptable thoughts and feelings activate defense mechanisms. These mechanisms then help to repress those thoughts at the unconscious level. Failure to keep them away from the conscious result in anxiety.

Panic attacks, according to the psychoanalytical school, result from an unsuccessful defense against anxiety-provoking impulses. Panic attacks often are reported as occurring out of the blue, which would seem to imply that there was no identifiable trigger event. Yet, theorists believe that thorough psychodynamic probing would reveal an underlying psychological reason for the panic attack. Patients with panic disorder have been found to have a higher incidence of stressful life events and are also reported to experience a great amount of distress following them. Research indicates that the cause of panic attacks is likely to involve the unconscious meaning of stressful events, and that panic attacks may be related to somatic-physiological factors triggered by psychological reactions.

Freud further suggested that when inner danger is projected onto the outer world it manifests itself as phobia. This, according to him, was the result of unresolved childhood Oedipal conflicts. As an adult, the individual is influenced by unresolved, incestuous sexual desires leading to anxiety and fear of castration. In phobic patients displacement is a typical and commonly used defense mechanism, with the unacceptable sexual conflict displaced from the person to seemingly unimportant situations or objects. The phobic object or situation may have a direct, associative connection with the primary source of conflict and may thus symbolize it (defense mechanism of symbolization).

Psychoanalytic theorists have suggested that, besides castration anxiety, phobias can result due to many other types of anxiety. For instance, separation anxiety and the loss of a parent play an important role in agoraphobia, whereas being alone in public places stimulates the childhood anxiety of abandonment, thereby triggering the panic attack. Trauma experienced due to separation in childhood may be so intense and pervasive that the child becomes an adult susceptible to anxieties.

For obsessive-compulsive disorder, the psychoanalytic viewpoint suggests a displacement activity which has the capacity to distract the person from essential concerns (*Salzman, 1995*). Freud explained the etiology of this disorder through defense mechanisms such as isolation, undoing and reaction formation. In the classical psychoanalytic theory, obsessive-compulsive disorder (earlier known as obsessive-compulsive neurosis) was due to regression from the Oedipal stage of development to the anal stage. When individuals feel threatened following the loss of a significant person's love in the Oedipal stage, they regress to the anal stage of psychosexual development which is characterized by ambivalent emotions. The reasons for this ambivalence are the inability to distinguish between sexual and aggressive drives, and the confusion caused by simultaneous feelings of love and hate towards the same person. The conflicting, opposing emotions manifest in "doing" and "undoing" behaviors. Thus, patients with obsessive-compulsive disorder may display extreme preoccupation with an act/image or a repetitive thought as, for example, with an act of cleanliness or a thought such as "I may push someone into a ditch" coming repeatedly into the mind much against the person's wishes. It has been suggested that disturbances and traumas experienced during the anal stage of development lead to such disorders in adulthood.

Post-traumatic and acute stress disorder are psychodynamically explained through the revival of childhood trauma, in that the ego resorts to defenses such as regression, denial and undoing in order to reduce the tension and anxiety caused by the revived memories of the trauma. Post-traumatic stress disorder is a symptom which wards off anxiety and thus gets reinforced.

Learning theory explanation for anxiety disorders

All behaviors are learned, and so also anxiety. This may have occurred either through modeling of faulty parental behaviors or through the process of classical conditioning. For instance, in panic disorder and agoraphobia, (two variants of anxiety disorders) a noxious element (panic reaction such as choking or feeling out of breath) occurs in conjunction with a neutral stimulus (taking the elevator to go to an upper or lower floor). The severity of the discomfort experienced causes panic and becomes associated with the neutral stimulus, leading the person to avoid this stimulus. Learning theory postulates that sensations associated with panic attack symptoms (palpitations, sweating, etc) can, by themselves, generate a panic disorder. Watson, a behaviorist, used the Pavlovian model of conditioned reflex in which anxiety resulted when a frightening stimulus occurred in the presence of a neutral one. When these two stimuli were paired on several occasions, over a period of time the neutral stimulus became the conditioned stimulus and acquired the capacity to provoke anxiety.

Operant conditioning, on the other hand, explains anxiety as a drive that impels the organism to do everything within reach to reduce or eliminate the distress associated with it. Through random, intermittent reinforcement, the individual learns that certain behaviors can help him avoid the anxiety-arousing source. Since avoidance behaviors are self-reinforcing due to their capacity to reduce anxiety, they become stable with repetition. Thus, phobias are avoidance behaviors learned to ward off anxiety.

Modeling is another mechanism through which a behavior is learned. In this technique, an attempt is made to associate the object/situation of phobia with the emotions that it evokes. Here, two things happen: (a) the subject, for example, a child may have observed the reaction of a significant person such as a parent who displays fear when he encounters a particular stimulus and escapes from the situation and (b) information transfer wherein the child may be told and warned repeatedly of the ways to escape from a threatening situation. This twin process of observation (of faulty behavior) and information transfer (incorrect/ misplaced information) serves, over a period of time, as a basis for instilling fear-arousing anxiety and avoiding the same.

The two processes described here are used to explain anxiety disorders. Social phobia is explained by behaviorists as occurring due to behavioral inhibition observed by children in their parents who, when encountering social situations, showed panic reactions. Children observe the parents avoiding such situations by panic reaction and model this behavior in their lives whenever they, in turn, encounter social situations. Such parents also fail to inculcate adequate social skills in their children and thus these children tend to show anxiety in social situations, leading to the development of a phobia in adulthood.

According to the behavioral school of thought, obsession is a result of conditioned stimuli, wherein a relatively neutral stimulus becomes associated with fear as a result of being paired with noxious or anxiety producing stimuli. Compulsions, on the other hand, are established when a person discovers that a certain act reduces the anxiety that comes with a particular, repetitive, noxious stimulus having a sexual or aggressive component. The moment the anxiety is reduced, the act that reduced anxiety gets reinforced and so whenever the noxious stimulus occurs, the act is resorted to. This ritualistic behavior becomes a sort of active avoidance strategy and is reinforced and maintained over a period. It is not always that an obsessive thought is accompanied by a compulsion, but an individual may reduce the anxiety associated with the unacceptable thought by thinking on a more "neutral" plane (e.g., a father who has incestuous thoughts may reduce his anxiety by thinking of killing others or himself).

Post-traumatic stress disorder can be explained through classical conditioning, where the trauma (unconditioned stimulus) of the stressor gets associated with the physical, emotional and mental reminders of the trauma (conditioned stimulus). Over a period of time, the patient develops a pattern of avoidance of both the unconditioned and conditioned stimulus. Cognitively he is unable to process or rationalize the trauma and its re-experience.

Behaviorists explain generalized anxiety disorder in terms of a learned incorrect, inaccurate perception of a threatening or dangerous stimulus. Since the perception is inadequate, it reduces the intensity of the dangerous stimulus. This is followed by a generalization of the perception to all events that are dangerous and threatening, making the individual pay attention only to the negative aspects of the situation. Naturally, this leads to a distorted and negative view of one's capacity to cope.

Biological explanation for anxiety disorder

Abnormalities in the brain structure and brain function are considered important biological causes of panic disorder. Studies have shown that both the peripheral and central nervous system dysregulation can cause panic disorder. The three major neurotransmitters viz., norepinephrine, serotonin and gamma aminobutynic acid (GABA) have been found to be associated with anxiety. There are certain panic-inducing substances called panicogens, such as sodium lactate and bicarbonate. Research studies on brain imaging have shown cortical atrophy in the right temporal lobe in panic disorder patients. Though available information is presently limited, these studies indicate a genetic basis for panic disorder and agoraphobia. Specific phobias, particularly related to the sight of blood, taking an injection and sustaining an injury are said to have a strong familial tendency, tracing back to biologically inherited dispositions.

Further evidence in this regard is based on the studies done on the first-degree relatives of persons with social phobia. Clinical trials of various drugs support the hypothesis that a dysregulation of serotonin is involved in the symptom formation of obsessions and compulsions. Serotonergic drugs were found to be more effective in treating these disorders compared to other drugs that act on the neurotransmitter systems. Brain imaging studies of patients with obsessive-compulsive disorders show stress-increased activity (metabolism and blood flow) in the frontal lobe and basal ganglia. These patients show a lower metabolic rate in basal ganglia and more white matter compared to the normal controls. Available data further indicates that obsessive-compulsive disorder has a genetic base. A genetic relationship between generalized anxiety disorder and major depressive disorder in women has also been demonstrated.

Sociocultural explanation for anxiety disorders

Every individual is born in a society and brought up within its sociocultural parameters. While family is the primary social unit that fulfills biological, psychological and social needs of an individual, the sociocultural milieu in which he is brought up instills in him the normative standards, values, attitudes and belief systems that he possesses.

The family is the keystone of a society and is important, both for the development of the individual as well for the enhancement of his strengths and assets. At the same time, it can also be responsible for the individual's vulnerabilities. Parents are the role models for the growing child and contribute to the development of his personality. Children who are given unconditional love and affection, care and nurturance develop within themselves the capacity to love, share and care for others. They also learn to value themselves on the basis of their own experience of being valued by the significant others.

When there is a negative role model, lack of nurturing, care, love and affection, the individual develops a negative self-image, high degree of insecurity and lack of confidence in himself. These may be manifested in varied types of psychological distress. Research has shown that there is a correlation between family pathology and psychiatric syndromes. Broken families, for example, frequently have been found to be associated with disorders such as sociopathic personality disorder, schizophrenia etc. Family deficiencies, particularly interpersonal and parental inadequacies, neurosis or psychosis in any or both parents, may lead to a poor interpersonal relationship between parents and children. This hinders care and nurturing which are essential for the healthy mental and physical growth of children. When, in a family, one or both parents suffer from some kind of mental disorder, the probability of their children developing similar behaviors is relatively high, not so much due to hereditary predisposition but due to modeling the parental behavior in different situations.

Negative child rearing may lead to the development of anxiety. If a parent, for instance, is inadequate or unable to portray him or herself in an appropriate gender or role model, it may cause uncertainty, confusion and social ineptness in the child. If a child is reared to feel that it will be loved or considered worthy only if it shows superior performance and achievement, it may keep it constantly under stress. In addition, if it is afraid that a slight fall from pre-set, high standards may result in reproach from parents, it will lead to anxiety, guilt and unhappiness.

Faulty communication within the family deprives children of opportunities to learn communication as a useful tool. This makes them anxious while attempting to deal with other people. Such anxiety can be overcome if there is love, support, and reassurance from the mother or the caregiver. Lack of such support or abandonment by the mother figure sets the basis for different types of anxiety disorders. Thus, negative early childhood experiences perpetuate feelings of anxiety and helplessness in persons which, in turn, may lead to distortion of all later relationships. Early fears of disapproval may be transferred from significant individuals to similar persons or authority figures in later life and accentuate already existing anxiety.

Anxiety disorders are caused by a large number of factors and experiences in a person's life, growth and development, and are explained by different theories and models. Based on these are different treatment strategies. For effective treatment, the clinician relies on various assessment strategies so as to be able to formulate an adequate diagnosis, and consequently, therapy. The following chapter discusses assessment strategies.

3
Assessment and Psychodiagnostics

A treatment plan for any disorder requires a thorough assessment of the patient, an understanding of the etiology of the disorder, the patient's personality and prognostic implications, including the psychodynamics, underlying the disorder. This implies obtaining information on different aspects of the disorder, symptomatology, the onset and intensity of the symptoms, premorbid personality, precipitating factors, interpersonal relationship dynamics and social support, as they all impinge upon the individual at the onset of symptoms. Kirk (1989) identified the aims of assessment as follows:

(1) To gain enough information to develop case conceptualization.
(2) To offer the patient useful understanding of what may be maintaining and causing his/her symptoms.
(3) To offer the patient a rationale for the therapy.
(4) To develop goals for therapy.

The essential stages in assessment are as follows:

Stage 1. Setting an agenda for assessment: This involves (a) Identifying and discussing the patient's symptoms, how he feels about visiting the clinic, and exploring the main problems and factors that maintain or exacerbate his symptoms (*b*) Description of the problems (somatic, cognitive, emotional responses, and behavior) (*c*) Identifying the situations, behaviors, mood, physiological factors, thoughts, other people and (*d*) Stresses that exacerbate maintain or reduce the symptom/problem.

Stage 2. Taking the Case History: This involves taking a detailed history of the problem, medical investigation, family history, treatment taken, relevant information regarding the problems the patient has had and the various belief systems of the patient which may be related to the symptoms and problems.

Stage 3. Mood and general functioning in the patient: This includes Mental Status Examination (MSE) and administration of psychological tests, if need be.

Stage 4. Assessment of interpersonal relationship: This involves ascertaining the type of relationship and support amongst family members as well as the patient's perception of himself and his reactions to others and vice-versa.

Stage 5. Conceptualization of the problem: This involves making a differential diagnosis and arriving at a correct answer. More specifically, it consists of synthesizing all the information obtained in the earlier stages and then combining the sociocultural influences to understand the symptamatology in the right perspective. This stage also includes developing goals for therapy.

While most information may be obtained from the patient, there are certain details that can be obtained only from relatives and others significant in the life of the patient. Psychology, psychiatry, and other professions in the field of mental health require talking to the patient to obtain the required information. From Freud to the neo-Freudians, learning theorists to the existentialists and the humanistic theorists, all therapists obtain information from the patient and his relatives through interviews, which are nothing but a particular form of talking. Interviewing requires complete and uninhibited cooperation from the patient as the diagnosis and treatment plans depend a great deal on how freely he talks. With the help of a relaxing and conducive atmosphere, the therapist encourages the patient to express his core thoughts and feelings deliberately establishing a relationship through which verbalization is facilitated. This free expression brings out much material repressed from childhood onward and is used to arrive at the correct diagnosis.

Assessment, as described earlier, provides a detailed and analytical psychological/psychiatric history of the patient's problems, a comprehensive view of his personality, and the underlying etiology of the disorder. Assessment is typically done through structured or unstructured interview, and is expected to cover the following areas:

- Early developmental history of the patient.
- Pre-morbid personality, i.e. personality of the patient before he fell ill.
- Experiences of success and failure in childhood, school, college and occupational life.
- Any hereditary disposition and genetic loading.
- Interpersonal and intra-familial relationships.
- Social interactions, peer interactions and relationships.
- Gender identity issues (if any).
- Development of sexual adaptation patterns.
- Identification of specific traumatic events.

During assessment, the therapist depends on (*a*) the responses of the patient to direct and indirect questioning (*b*) therapist's observation of the patient (*c*) the impression gained by the clinician on the basis of the patient's non verbal responses, such as mood, facial expression, posture, gesture, and manner of relating.

In addition, the therapist may prefer to use the standard procedure of mental status examination (MSE) which is partly based on his own observation and partly deduced from the answers to specific questions. Besides these two basic assessment strategies, the clinician may use psychological tests where the responses of the patient constitute a valuable source of information. Projective tests such as the Rorschach Test, Thematic Apperception Test (TAT), personality tests and neuro-psychological tests, are some of the major tools used for diagnostic and differential diagnostic purposes. Other psychological tests are also used for assessing specific sensory and motor deficits and sensory integration. Tests supplement and clarify information obtained in the interview and facilitate assessment of particular personality functions, the nature and extent of psychopathology, the intellectual potential of the patient and the presence of organic brain damage, if any. These, when synthesized with other information, help in understanding the psychodynamics and prognostic implications of the disorder.

Symptoms of various disorders are characterized by disturbances at many levels of psychological functioning. It is therefore important to consider the behavioral parameters that are most vulnerable to disruption by the disorder and the consequent psychological functioning. Assessment strategies are designed to bring to light the different psychopathological manifestations and behavioral features which point towards specific vulnerability, and the etiology and psychodynamics of the particular disorder. All these facilitate the planning of appropriate treatment strategies and also show the clinician the patient's potential for constructive change and growth, essential prerequisites for starting therapy. As discussed earlier, interviewing the patient is an essential stage before taking him up for testing. This requires the therapist to adhere to certain important principles and possess of certain skills. These have been elucidated in the following section.

Interviewing: Principles and Techniques

Interview is a purposeful and deliberately planned conversation between the therapist and the patient and others concerned or closely associated with the life of the patient. The therapist initiates the interview and, in order to obtain the needed information, strives to establish a good working relationship between himself and the patient. It is this relationship which is the core of the interviewing and therapeutic processes that follow. In a number of cases, this specially established relationship itself becomes sufficient to reduce the severity of the patient's symptoms.

The development of an effective working relationship depends on the rapport, that is the spontaneous, conscious feeling of harmonious responsiveness on part of both patient and therapist. Such a rapport promotes constructive therapeutic processes and implies mutual trust between patient and therapist. This relationship emerges as a result of the therapist (*a*) accepting the patient as he is (*b*) treating him with dignity and respect (*c*) considering him as a person of worth (*d*) being non-judgmental regarding all aspects of his behavior (*e*) giving due recognition his assets and (*f*) ensuring confidentiality of the information revealed by him.

In an effective interview, the patient's viewpoints are heard and listened to, and unconditionally accepted by a professional expert. The patient experiences being treated without any preconceived notions, being given importance as a person, and, above all, being understood by the expert. All these act, in combination, as a great source of comfort to the patient. A related aspect is that, even when the patient behaves negatively the therapist does not show any disapproval but indicates acceptance of such behavior too. For the therapist, these negative behaviors are of great importance as they are a replay of the patient's earlier attitude towards his own doctors, therapists, parents, teachers, and significant others. Such acceptance by the therapist facilitates uninhibited and free expression of feelings and emotions on part of the patient.

At this point in the interview process, verbalizing his emotions and feelings makes the patient feel less burdened and stressed. The therapist, on his part, continuously evaluates the relationship and uses it to direct the interview towards gaining a better insight into the psychodynamics of the patient's problems. This further facilitated by his understanding the problem from the patient's viewpoint as well as his own view. The therapist's role is not to take over the patient's problem, but to enhance his skills and help him develop the ability to tackle it by his own efforts.

During interview, problems might arise within the relationship itself but if the patient is convinced that the therapist is genuinely interested in his problems, he is likely to continue with the sessions and remain willing to talk. The therapist must ensure that no issue that is important to the patient is avoided or missed, so that the interview is able to achieve the purpose for which it was initiated.

While some patients might come to the therapist for parental type of guidance, a few might expect a magical cure. Sometimes, a patient comes to the therapist after being compelled by family members, and/or friends. If a patient is sent against his wishes, he may show anger, and be unreceptive and inhibited. The therapist has to use tact and understand the patient's resistance, anger and inhibition. By putting him at ease, free, uninhibited expression of problems and feelings is facilitated. The understanding and acceptance that the clinician shows not only encourages the patient to express his innermost feelings but also to answer questions freely and frankly. A knowledge of the psychodynamics underlying the problem helps the therapist understand the various conflicts experienced by the patient and the causes for his behavior.

Duration of the interview

Interviews should not last longer than an hour, although in some cases they may be prolonged. Since the ultimate aim of an interview is to help the patient express himself, acquire an understanding of his behavior and overcome symptoms, attitudes etc., more than one interview session may be required. Very long interviews exhaust both patient and therapist and, at times, may drift off into areas irrelevant to the therapeutic process or patient's problem. It is for the therapist to direct and control the interview in such a manner that it is possible to end the session within an hour, plus or minus fifteen minutes, and also decide on the next appointment.

"Beginning where the patient is"

In guiding the interview the therapist allows for uninterrupted, free expression of thoughts and feelings and lets the patient tell his story in his own way. When the patient has a disorder the interviewer focusses on the symptoms. If, however, the patient himself starts with a topic of his concern the therapist focusses his attention there and moves on to other aspects gradually. Since gaps can always be filled up later, the therapist considers it important to listen to the patient and encourage him to expand on his thoughts and bring up all relevant issues for discussion. Not only does the therapist listen but he also pays attention to both what the patient says as well as what he omits or avoids. It is important to remember not to immediately challenge any of the patient's dogmatic or emotionally charged statements. In fact, these should be used to further explore what he actually wants to convey and what underlies the statements. The clinician keeps in mind the need to encourage patients to discuss, at their own level, the advantages and disadvantages involved in dealing with a problem in a certain way so that they can learn about possible courses of action.

Dealing with resistance during interview

Whenever there is resistance on the part of patient, the questioning techniques have to be modified. Tactful questioning, which does not contradict the patient's concept of self would bring a response without resistance. In interviews, leading questions and interpretive comments should be avoided except in rare situations, as these may damage the patient's self image. In addition, the therapist should not try to influence the patient with his own preconceived notions or theories as these are of no relevance to him. The questions should be such that they lead to an analysis of the development of the symptoms, so that the patient can be helped to plan an adequate and effective strategy to handle his problems.

Directing the interview

The conversation during the interview should be guided so as to avoid sounding like a prosecution by an attorney. The therapist should be constantly aware of the purpose of each session and direct the interview towards that end. Simple explanations and praise may be used to obtain information as well as to alleviate anxiety. The therapist should avoid the use of slang and technical jargon. Moral, dictatorial, prejudicial or punitive statements should also be avoided.

Probing during interview

While probing is essential, there are occasions when the patient may not be ready to discuss certain problems. In such situations, the therapist should be sensitive to the feelings of the patient and not insist on continuing with the topic. This avoids embarrassment to the patient, make him more comfortable, and encourages him to take up the same issue, when ready, in later sessions. The therapist also should avoid giving interpretation in the initial stages as it may cause considerable anxiety to the patient, though clarifications may be provided to help him think objectively and clearly.

Ending interviews

Ending each interview session in the right manner is important so that the patient continues to attend subsequent sessions. An abrupt ending to a session giving the patient the feeling that the therapist being overly conscious of time and should be avoided. Ending an interview smoothly and comfortably can be accomplished if the therapist summarizes briefly what transpired during the session and what could be discussed in the next one. The therapist should also help the patient fix his next appointment.

Interview with family members

While the techniques of interviewing elucidated here have to be carefully followed, an interview with a patient suffering from an anxiety disorder requires the therapist to focus on the thoughts and environmental stressors that precipitate or exacerbate anxiety in him. When stressors are not evident, careful and detailed investigation through projective tests may be essential in order to get to the roots of the anxiety. Restraining forces have to be gradually overcome, and an analysis should be made of the current situation within and without the family that evokes anxiety. In many cases, the original stimuli that caused anxiety might have been projected symbolically on others and, by being sensitive to this aspect, the therapist could delineate the causes. Use of dreams and other relevant information that emerge during the interview may indicate to the therapist interpersonal relationships and self-regulated problems. A chronology of the sequence of events related to the main problem helps unravel the underlying causes as well as to exclude some explanations that may be otherwise applicable. Success in such endeavors depends on the therapist's skill in interviewing the patient and his family, and the type of professional relationship that has been established. Other methods include guided discovery, where the questions are put forth in such a manner that the patient discovers new ways of seeing the situation rather than merely answering in the affirmative or negative. Given in Box 3.1 is a brief summary of some of the communication skills that are needed by the interviewer to facilitate the process of gathering information. These are essential for patients suffering from anxiety disorders but can be used anywhere that such information is needed.

Box 3.1: Various kinds of communication skills that are used in interviewing

Skills	Definition	Example
• Acceptance of the client's statement	A verbal statement or gesture which communicates interest on part of the therapist towards the client.	"Uh ... oh" "Well" Nods head
• Non-evaluative description of what is transpiring in the session	Neutral expression by the therapist regarding the current situation.	"It seems that the statement made by me has upset you"
• Mirroring the client's statement	A summarized statement by the therapist that repeats what the client has said and thereby reflects back to him what has been said.	"So what you are saying is that you were angry when she walked out on you" *(Box 3.1 continued)*

• Appreciation of the client	A statement or gesture on part of the therapist which shows positive evaluation of the clients behaviour.	"You have done a good job of maintaining this thought recorder"
• The inquiring approach	An expression of inquiry to elicit information.	"Tell me what is it that you can do to help your son out"
• Statements that show disapproval or condescend the client (*to be avoided*)	A statement that expresses judgement on part of the therapist.	"That was very silly" "You are weird"

An excerpt from an interview session is reproduced in Box 3.2 to give an idea of some of the intricacies involved in interviewing. The therapist is in conversation with a patient suffering from claustrophobia with panic attacks while in an elevator. The content of the patient's anxiety within the contextual framework (here, being in the elevator) highlights, among other things, how the right questions can elicit the needed information.

Box 3.2: Transcript of an interview session

Transcript	Remarks
C "There are three elevators in the building where my office is located. I am usually able to get elevators which are not stuffed with people. However, on that day two lifts were out of order and I had no option but to use the lift which was crowded. It is not possible to climb stairs to the twentieth floor where my office is."	
T "How did you feel while getting on to the elevator?"	Therapist focusses on sensations
C "The small elevator had about a dozen people, I wondered how I would fit in and suddenly I stopped as the liftman asked me to step in. He seemed a little irritable as I was taking an inordinate amount of time. I stepped in and my throat went dry."	This is the imagined fear associated when the individual's perception of the situation is faulty and distorted. This imagined fear is also effective in producing or completing the panic attack.

(Box 3.2 continued) |

T "As of now are you feeling the same sensations as you did then."

C "My throat feels a little tight and mouth is dry."

Therapist offers a glass of water and then continues.

T "Are you feeling better now, would you like to continue now as to what happened next?" (client nods).

Therapist displays concern for the client rather than bulldozing him.

C "Like I said, there were about ten people. I entered, the door closed and the elevator moved up. The elevator stopped on the next floor. Couple of people entered. I felt panicky and wanted to scream 'why do these people keep coming in?' but my tongue seem stuck and no voice came out."

Because of the therapist concern, the client perceives himself to be safe and continues.

T "You wanted to scream at the people who entered after you but your voice seemed to be lost."

Therapist rephrases and reflects what the client has said. Rephrasing is important as it helps the client to stay focussed and encourages him to give further information.

C "Yes, that is right. I wanted to shout out but could not."

T "And you were standing next to someone?"

Eliciting more details with a precise question.

C "Yes, I was between two young men who seemed to know each other as they were talking to each other but did not seem to notice my predicament. I clutched on to my briefcase and prayed that it would reach my floor fast."

T "Hmm., Hmm, what happened then?"

A comment with little manifest content but enough to persuade the client to carry on.

C "But suddenly the elevator came to a halt, everyone started talking all at once. Some were shouting, one said that the elevator had stopped because of overload. I could not see anything. I

(Box 3.2 continued)

wished that there were small peepholes so that I could see what was outside."

T "Just stop here for a minute—how are you feeling? Comfortable enough to go on further?"

Finding out how the patient felt when he is re-experiencing the panic attack in the therapeutic session.

T "You were feeling shut in?"

C "Yes, I felt shut in. I sat down as I thought 'I am going to have a heart attack'."

T "You felt you would have a heart attack as you were shut in?"

The therapist re-phrases the clients feelings and statement. This encourages patient to continue.

C (a moment later) "Yes, I spoke to one of the young man next to me to take my mind off the situation."

Client uses distraction.

T "I want you to imagine the situation once again as vividly as possible...you enter the lift which is full of people...more people come, you are surrounded by people. You cannot get any breath of fresh air; you look for a peephole...you want to get out but cannot. How do you feel about it?"

Therapist tries to strengthen the image and emotions to bring out the thoughts.

(T: Therapist; C: Client)

Thus a skilled therapist could, through tactful questioning and handling of the responses during interview sessions, help patients verbalize their feelings, anxiety and apprehension, as has been seen in the excerpt from an interview.

There are, however, many times when even detailed and tactful interviews may not be able to elicit responses from patients with high resistance. When the therapist encounters such resistance, psychological tests could be used to elicit the required information. This procedure essentially has three stages:

(1) Setting an agenda for assessment.
(2) Selection of an appropriate test.

(3) Scoring, interpretation and relating the test results with the patient's problem.

Psychological Tests (Paper and Pencil Type)

Psychological tests could be viewed as microscopes or X-rays, as these reflect certain selected performances of the person in real life. Different tests yield different information and provide new insights into certain psychological aspects involved in the manifestation of symptoms. The tests access information that is not available through direct interviewing, as for instance, in differentiating adequately between the highest performance level and that of the level of actual effective potential of a patient. With the help of psychological tests it is possible to make such differentiation. The norms of every standardized test enable the therapist to evaluate the performance of an individual in terms of a particular population on which the test has been standardized.

Psychological tests vary in their degree of reliability and their uses in different settings. The application and interpretation of certain tests require a long period of training and hence may not be used by many therapists. Projective tests, for instances, specially the Rorschach and the TAT are among the more difficult ones to score, analyze and interpret, and require psychologists well trained in their use. On the other hand, the paper–pencil tests are relatively easy and eliminate the influence of the examiner in both administration and interpretation. But there are certain tests, such as tests of intelligence, where the norms may not be applicable even for the population under consideration and so have to be interpreted with the greatest caution. Some of the psychological tests, both Indian and foreign, can be considered under the following six categories:

(1) Intelligence tests
(2) Personality tests (paper and pencil)
(3) Projective Personality tests
(4) Free Drawing tests
(5) Neuro-psychological tests (unless organicity is suspected, these tests are not used in anxiety disorder cases)

(6) Rating Scales (examples, Brief Psychiatric Rating Scale, Global Assessment Scale and Observation Scale for inpatient evaluation).

In assessing anxiety, self-report methods, questionnaires, protocol analyses, situational ratings, self-monitoring etc., are commonly used. In addition, contrived behavioral avoidance tests, interpersonal performance test, measurement of physical reactions, such as heart rate, electrodermal rate, and respiration are used in anxiety disorder. It may be pointed out that there are different scales for different anxiety disorders. While deciding which test is to be used for assessment, the psychologist must deliberate on (a) rationale for testing (b) the choice of the test and (c) the number of tests to be administered. No test should be administered without a clear rationale and an idea of what it would yield in terms of the required information. In a few selective cases or disorders, the psychologist might use three or four tests as no single test provides a clear picture of the underlying conflicts or problems.

Another aspect to be kept in mind while using psychological tests is that these should not be used as a routine, for example, if during the interview it becomes clear that the individual possesses average intelligence, it is preferable to proceed with the other tests needed, rather than administering an intelligence test. Similarly, if brain damage or organicity is suspected, it is better to straight away administer neuropsychological tests rather than any others. A clear decision needs to be taken on the use of appropriate psychological tests, based on a thorough analysis of the patient's history. Some psychological tests used in clinical settings to diagnose and for the differential diagnosis of anxiety disorders are given in Box 3.3.

It is worth reiterating that appropriate and adequate assessment are important pre-requisites for effective clinical work. In recent times, the behavioral approach to assessment is being widely recommended. By emphasizing a triple-response modality, namely, overt behavior, cognitive components and physiological activity, a comprehensive account of the patient's problems is

Box 3.3: Some psychological tests used in clinical settings

Name of tests	Author & Year	Uses
Projective Personality Tests		
The Rorschach Test	H. Rorschach (1951)	An effective tool for differential diagnosis. Provides clear indicators of personality traits.
Thematic Apperception Test	H.A. Murray (1943)	Delineates intrapsychic conflicts, ungratified needs and obstacles from the environment.
Thematic Apperception Test (Indian Adaptation)	L.P. Mehrotra (1992)	-do-
Incomplete Sentences Blank	J.B. Rotter and J.E. Rafferty (1950)	-do-
Free Drawing Tests		
Draw a person Test	F.L. Goodenough (1926)	Provides information on personality factors and traits.
Kinetic Family Drawing Test	R. Burns & S. Kaufman (1970)	Provides information on interpersonal relationships amongst different family members and the subject.
Tests that Measure Anxiety		
Social Avoidance Distress	D. Watson & R. Friend (1969)	28 item scales with True/False responses to identify situations that are socially distressing for the individual.
Social Interaction Self-Statement Test	C. Glass et al (1982)	Measures adaptive and maladaptive thought content in social phobia.

(Box 3.3 continued)

Name of tests	Author & Year	Uses
Social Phobia and Anxiety Inventory	S.M. Turner et al (1989)	Subject rates his subjective and behavioral psychological responses in social settings and Agoraphobia.
Social Situations Interaction Test	P.A. Mersch et al (1989)	It has four vignettes with male and female confederates to help measure social anxiety.
State-Trait Anxiety Inventory	C. Spielberger et al (1983)	Measures general anxiety disorder.
Subjective Limits of Discomfort Scale Test	J. Wolpe (1973)	Self-reports about fear intensity associated with imaging.
Pleasant and Unpleasant Events Schedule Scale	L. Teri & P.M. Lewinsohn (1982)	Checklist in which behavioral activities are rated for frequency pleasantries and implementation.
Yale–Brown Obsessive Compulsive Scale	W. Goodman et al (1989a, b)	Has five items of obsessive thinking and compulsive behavior with a rating on 0–4 point scale of severity.
Leyton Obsessional Inventory	J. Cooper (1970)	Card sort procedure in 46 items evaluates obsessive symptoms and 23 items of obsessive personality tests.
Irrational Belief Test	R.G. Jones (1968)	Evaluates the cognitive level of the beliefs.
Interactional Behaviors and Pattern Questionnaire	L.J. Roberts and K.E. Leonard (1992)	Assesses the frequency of four types of Interactional sequences arranged with engagement and avoidance behaviors.
Fear Survey Schedule	J. Wolpe & P.J. Lang (1964)	Fear intensity ratings about commonly feared objects.
Naturalistic Behavioral Avoidance Test	R.P. Mattick & L. Peters (1988)	Assesses social phobia
The Compulsive Activity Checklist (CAC)	I.M. Marks et al (1977)	Assesses through 37 items the degree of interference by obsession in functioning.

(Box 3.3 continued)

Name of tests	Author & Year	Uses
Four Systems of Anxiety Questionnaire (FSQA)	F. Koskal & K.G. Power (1990)	A self-report measure of four aspects of anxiety—physiological, cognitive, behavioral and psychological aspects.
Fear Questionnaire	I.M. Marks & A.M. Mathews (1979)	A brief self-rating scale which assess the degree of phobia.
Penn State Worry Questionnaire	T.J. Meyer et al (1990)	Assesses and quantifies the worry behavior in Generalized Anxiety Patients.
Beck Anxiety Inventory (BAI)	A. Beck et al (1988)	Evaluates cognitive, somatic and behavioral manifestations of anxiety.
Automatic Thoughts Questionnaire—Negative	S.D. Hollon & P.C. Kendall (1980)	A 30-item scale and self-report instrument, it measures the frequency of negative statements regarding oneself.
Anxiety Index Scale	A.S. Patel (1956)	Provides a measure of anxiety.
The Anxiety Scale	D.N. Srivastava & G. Tiwari (1973)	Measures manifest anxiety in individuals.
Srivastava Anxiety Scale	Ramji & Bina Srivastava (1988)	Provides a measure of anxiety.
Self Analysis Questionnaire	H. Badami & C. Badami (1988)	Measures the perceived level of anxiety amongst subjects.
Dutt Personality Inventory (DPI)	N.K. Dutt (1966)	For clinical diagnosis and measuring anxiety.
Sinha's Anxiety Scale (Self Analysis Form)	D. Sinha (1968)	Provides a measure of anxiety and locates the forms and dimensions in which anxiety may express itself.
Medico-Psychological Questionnaire (MPQ)	Bharath Raj (1992)	Provides for making differential diagnosis within subcategories of neurosis,

(Box 3.3 continued)

Name of tests	Author & Year	Uses
		namely, hysteria, neurasthenia, anxiety neurosis, reactive depression and obsessive-compulsive disorder.
PGI-Health Questionnaire N-I	S.K. Verma, N.N. Wig, D. Preshad (1985)	Provides differential diagnosis for anxiety, depression and hysteria.

obtained. A variety of techniques ranging from standardized empirical measures and projective tests to limited idiosyncratic subjective evaluation may be used to assess anxiety. Specific assessment measures for anxiety broadly include (*a*) Self-report Measures (*b*) Motoric Behavior Assessment and (*c*) Physiological Assessment.

Self-report measures

Spielberger (1972) pointed out that, "... If an individual reports that he feels anxious, frightened or apprehensive, this introspective report defines an anxiety state" (p. 30). The central feature of such measures is the acceptance and acknowledgement of a person's subjective distress as being integral to anxiety. Self-report measures elicit information at two levels:

(1) Reports of physiological activity, motoric responses and cognitions (examples, "Do you get 'pins and needles'?" "Does your heart pound?" "Do you have self-critical thoughts?", etc.)
(2) Reports of a person's subjective experiences indicate the interplay of the individual's expectations, values, and cognitive sets (example, "Do you feel anxious and tense?" "Do you fear approaching a stranger at a social gathering?", etc.)

There are two types of self-report measures: self-monitoring and anxiety scales and inventories.

SELF-MONITORING

Kazdin (1974) defined it as the ongoing observation of one's own behavior. It refers to the keeping of records by the patient, of various aspects of his own behavior. These may range from simple frequency counts to more elaborate ones in which details of the situational antecedents, consequent behavior and affect are maintained. This form of assessment can assist in the measurement of the frequency and intensity of the problem and may yield valuable information about factors that reinforce a particular behavior. It also strengthens the collaborative nature of the therapeutic endeavor. Such self-monitoring forms can be devised and tailored to meet the specific needs of the client. It is important, on part of the clinician, to explain to the client the purpose of such a form and how the information provided will be of use to the therapeutic alliance. Box 3.4 provides one example of a self-monitoring record which can be used to identify events that are anxiety provoking, and the accompanying cognitions, behaviors and consequences. In this example, the "fear thermometer" of Walk (1956), which is a scale of 0–10, has been used to measure anxiety.

Another kind of self-monitoring form is the thought recorder, that helps the patient to highlight the thoughts associated with his anxiety and fear. The thought recorder provides the therapist with information underlying the anxiety experienced by the patient. The clinician uses this information in therapy to help the patient become aware of the problem and educate him on the dynamics underlying the symptoms. A facsimile of the thought recorder is given in Boxes 3.5 and 3.6.

In certain cases where the patient does not require such a structured form to report or keep track of various activities, he may be asked to maintain a diary. This is a personal record giving an intimate account of his personal experiences and related positive and negative feelings. The patient records all the situational antecedents, behaviors and thoughts that he experiences in anxiety-provoking situations and their effect on his activities and interactions. Such self-monitored information is valuable in assessing the nature and degree of the problem and in understanding its

Box 3.4: Anxiety-monitoring form

In the space below, record the times you thought you may encounter objects and situations that worry you.
. . . .
. . . .

Describe
- the time and place
- the situation
- what were you thinking
- what you did
- what followed after
- rate your anxiety on the following scale

0	1	2	3	4	5	6	7	8	9	10
No anxiety				*Moderate anxiety*					*Extreme anxiety*	

Date . . . .
Time . . . .
Place . . . .
Situation . . . .
Thought . . . .
Behavior . . . .
Consequences . . . .
Anxiety experienced . . . .

Box 3.5: The thought recorder (a blank record)

Situational antecedents	Behavior and feelings	Automatic thoughts (images)
Who, what, where and when is anxiety triggered.	• What did you do in the situation (fight–flight–freeze) • What sensation/feelings did you experience?	What were the thoughts and images in your mind during that situation?

Box 3.6: The thought recorder
(a filled-in record of a person who fears flying)

Situational antecedents	Behavior and feelings	Automatic thoughts (images)
Waiting for the plane to take off.	• *Behavior* "I had this strong urge to get off the plane." • *Sensations/feelings* "My mouth was dry and chest was tight as if it would burst open. I felt dread as the sign to fasten seat belts was flashed".	1. "What if the plane develops a engine snag—I will be gone forever." 2. "What if I have a panic attack, the other passengers will laugh at me." *Image* "I am going to have a heart attack, I am clutching my chest and I am drenched in sweat and have turned white."

complexity. It also provides an account of the individual's reactions to the past, present and future events. Valuable information can be gleaned about the patient's perception of the significant others in his life, in terms of how they contribute, maintain or exacerbate his symptoms. Any information on the social and family support the patient perceives as available to him and the sources of security and safety can be effectively used in treatment.

ANXIETY SCALES AND INVENTORIES

Anxiety Scales and Inventories constitute another method of obtaining self-report data. These inventories measure either trait anxiety, state anxiety or situation specific anxiety. Trait anxiety refers to a general and stable disposition in an individual to become anxious over a wide range of stimuli. Typical prototype tests ask the testee how they feel and act in various situations and the overall scores obtained on the inventory reflect the degree of anxiety. State anxiety is conceptualized as a transitory anxiety response which is situationally determined and can vary from moment to moment (Spielberger, 1972). State anxiety can usually be ascertained by such tests as they have items that ask patients how they feel right at the moment or how they felt at some immediately preceding point.

The third subtype of such inventories/scales are situation-specific devices which measure anxiety in circumscribed situations. The Test Anxiety Questionnaire (*Mandler and Sarason, 1952*) is used for assessing examination anxiety. Usually, information from such tests acts as basal data that reflect any alleviation or reduction in the anxiety symptoms since the start of intervention strategies.

Although widely used in clinical settings, self-reports are not bereft of problems. Terms such as fear, anxiety, apprehension etc. are used in a relative sense by the patient and are, therefore, subject to variable interpretation. The degree or intensity of distress that qualifies as anxiety varies from person to person. Terms used to describe frequency of attacks—such as "often", "sometimes", "seldom"—have different meanings for different people and their usage may not be completely accurate. In a number of tests, the wording is not specific and, consequently, leads to a loose, generally idiosyncratic translation of what is being asked rather than what the patient actually experiences and feels. Another problem with self-reports is that the information provided is based on the clients' observation of his own behavior and, therefore, bound to involve his own biases and subjectivity. The information provided may be conjectural and, therefore, inaccurate. Despite these shortcomings, self-reports, if maintained by the patient taking all necessary precautions and following the therapist's instructions, can be reliable and valuable in arriving at a correct diagnosis and planning a proper treatment intervention.

Motoric behavior assessment

The underlying feature of motoric behavior assessment is the direct observation of the patient's behavior in the natural environment. For a number of reasons, it is rather difficult to collect data from naturalistic observation for clinical work. Therefore, situational contexts under the clinician's control are created for behavioral observation. The creation of these situations for assessing anxiety is based on the assumption that a sample of the behavior obtained under such conditions is representative of the patient's behavior in real-life situations. To give an example, while dealing with a phobic patient in the laboratory (or clinician's chamber), the clinician presents a stimulus (a snake, a ladder to climb etc.) and notes the motoric behavior of the patient (trembling, shaking, quickening of the breath), as well as his motoric response in terms of distance (did the patient run away shrieking or push the stimulus away or shrink from it). The clinician may also note the time taken by the patient to react to the phobic stimulus. In another instance, if the patient has social phobia (speech anxiety) the subject may be requested to interact with confederates of the clinician who, in turn, rate the motoric behavior of the subject. Both, physiological effects (sweating, restlessness, shaking) and performance disruption (stammering, speech blocks, omissions and repetitions) of anxiety, are noted. These measures are analyzed by the clinician to arrive at the level of anxiety in the client.

Physiological assessment

Since the arousal of the sympathetic autonomic nervous system is known to be dominant during anxiety, measurement of physiological arousal is viewed as an integral part of anxiety assessment. These physiological responses often correspond to the somatic complaints reported by the individual while experiencing high levels of anxiety, for instance, increased muscle tone manifesting as headaches, reduced gastrointestinal activity leading to constipation, dry mouth, increased cardiac output and heart rate perceived as a "pounding heart".

Physiological measurement is a reliable index of anxiety as it is free from subject bias. Clinicians consider, for example, that heart rate is a more valid and useful gauge of anxiety than self-reports, as it is measured by objective methods making it a reliable input during assessment and therapy. However, research comparing self-reports and physiological measures of anxiety during treatment with flooding technique have indicated that self-report was found to reduce the length of the session by approximately 75 per cent (*Andrasik, Turner and Ollendick, 1980*).

Certain disadvantages of physiological measurement include the need for expertise in psychophysiology and for cumbersome, expensive equipment.

While motoric behavior and physiological assessment appear to overlap considerably, both these methods when used together on a patient according to his symptomatology, provide a more adequate picture than when used simply. In motoric behavior assessment, autonomic nervous system responses are not monitored. A situation created and the patient is put into it and his overt, observable reactions are recorded in detail. Here, there is no specific score or measurement of the exact amount of emitted sweat, say, as in a physiological assessment of anxiety. When the latter technique is used, no situation is created. Anxiety is measured as and when it is aroused, which may be immediately after the event or a little later. One of the problems faced in such an assessment is that the reactions evoked by a particular event may not be immediately measurable. This is because the event may have passed by the time the equipment to measure the physiological parameters is assembled. Between these two methods, even though a certain amount of subjectivity is involved, motoric behavior assessment appears to be more the practical.

In addition, certain projective tests may also be used in assessment of different anxiety disorders.

Psychological Tests (Projective)

Projective tests present certain stimuli whose meanings are not immediately obvious and can be interpreted according to the subject's own perception and understanding. In other words, the stimulus is ambiguous and this forces the patient to project his own needs into the test situation. Such tests have no right or wrong answers. Instead, the person to whom the test is administered has to give meaning to the stimulus in accordance with his inner needs, drives, abilities, and defenses. Examples of such tests are the Rorschach Test, the Thematic Apperception Test, the Sentence Completion Test and Draw A Person Test. A brief description and indicators of anxiety for each of these tests are presented here.

Thematic apperception test (TAT)

This projective test essentially helps to delineate the underlying intra-psychic conflicts causing the symptoms. The test provides the clinician information on the ungratified needs of the patient, the major areas of conflicts, the environmental pressures and the obstacles that hinder the gratification of his needs. TAT, though not very helpful in differential diagnosis, can provide the clinician with certain important indicators that help facilitate an adequate treatment and therapy plan. For instance, the most characteristic response of obsessive-compulsive disorder to TAT cards includes arguing back and forth without making a definite decision or judgement. Obsessive individuals take considerable care not to be misunderstood, and tend to repeat themselves and explain not only their themes but also how they happened to think of them, why they thought of a particular story etc., hoping that this dispels any impression that they may have created on the therapist. The essential feature in the TAT protocol of hysterical disorder patients is their ineffectually striving for emotional relationships that are beyond their capacity. The desire to avoid anxiety and disappointment is so strong that it leads to a certain degree of psychological blindness.

The Rorschach test

The Rorschach signs of anxiety and insecurity, as opposed to signs of a balanced personality structure, focus on systematized and unsystematized anxiety. While systematized anxiety produces a neurotic defense system, expressed through marked changes in the personality structure of a hysterical or compulsive disorder, unsystematized anxiety can be seen in free floating anxiety, in the plain diffusion response (K such as smoking, whirling water, etc.). The physical qualities of the shading effects reflect the corresponding qualities of the inner life of the subject, that is haziness and fogginess created by free-floating anxiety. The K and k indicate a flight from the more sensuous shading effects and whenever these are high, it is indicative of the fact that so much of anxiety and guilt are aroused that the subject is not able to handle them. The "k" indicates an intellectual attempt to de-personalize or objectify the haziness expressed in k, as obtained in responses such as X-rays pictures, maps etc., in all of which the subject appears to be intellectualizing his/her anxiety.

Shading shock, which indicates anxiety, may occur in conjunction with color shock or by itself. Anxiety can also take the form of evasiveness, where the subject merely describes rather than interprets the card, the lines and dots, or he may give responses such as "islands", "bones", "peninsula" etc. In a person suffering from neurotic disorder, color seems to constitute a new and catastrophic situation, which requires a shift in behavior pattern. The criteria to determine color shock indicating anxiety in the Rorschach are:

- Delayed reaction time
- Exclamations
- Comments made by the subject indicating anxiety, tension or stress
- Decline in total number of responses to all the color (chromatic) cards *vis-à-vis* the non-color cards
- Impoverished content
- Rejection of cards

Briefly stated, the classical signs of anxiety in the Rorschach response are:

- An initial delay in the production of a meaningful interpretation of a new stimulus.
- Failure to give any response to a Rorschach card or to all cards, which indicates the highest degree of anxiety or shock.
- The color shock, associated with the color red, indicating neurotic ambivalence regarding emotions towards others.
- Color shock responses indicating anxiety in a person, in addition to a tendency to blame others for his own frustrations.
- Dark shading shock, associated with anxious and depressed states and feelings of inferiority, as well as blaming oneself for one's frustrations.

The classic response to the Rorschach of an obsessive-compulsive disorder patient would be:

- To perceive the blot well and to suggest a sharply conceived form to fit the blot area.
- To note spontaneously and to know the discrepancy between the blots, their shapes or color as well as those of the imagined objects.
- To be right about the discrepancies and to steadfastly keep in mind both the sensation of the blot and the image of the object while comparing them with each other.
- Limiting freedom of action in the human or animal responses indicates difficulty in making vital decisions because of extreme obsessiveness about taking the correct decision.
- When movement and color responses are about equal in number and there is dark shading shock, the character structure of the person is likely to be obsessive-compulsive.

Patients suffering from hysterical disorders produce very few anatomical responses and are not concerned about the adequacy of their test response. Their perceptiveness is also found to be limited.

The Rorschach test excels as an aid in making neuro-psychiatric diagnosis, which more frequently helps in understanding the syndromes. However, diagnosis based only on the Rorschach protocol may not be adequate and it is important to consider the information obtained from the Rorschach test along with detailed case history of the patient in order to arrive at the correct diagnosis.

Draw a person test (DAP)

DAP was developed by Florence Goodenough in 1926 as an intelligence scale that was based on the drawing of a man. With time, clinicians came to realize that although DAP was supposed to be a test of intelligence, the drawings also tapped a variety of personality variables. Encouraging the subjects to tell stories based on their drawing helped in getting much-needed information about the individual and his/her problems. Although drawings are generally used with children, they can also be used with adults to obtain an insight into intrapsychic conflicts. The DAP is simple and easy to administer, does not require any external stimulus or structure, has few age and intelligence limitations and often yields a great deal of information regarding self-concept, personality style, orientation and conflict areas. In addition, the DAP has a therapeutic value as the act of drawing allows for catharsis. Interpretation of drawings is done broadly at two levels (a) Structure and (b) Content.

Structural interpretation includes size, pencil pressure, strokes, detailing and placement of drawings, erasure and shading.

SIZE

It has been reported the average size of the drawing of a human figure on an A4 sheet is about seven inches and deviations in size must be considered relative to the size of paper used. The size of the drawing is indicative of the self-esteem of a person, for instance, a person who feels inadequate and inferior usually tends to make a tiny figure. Others may draw on the whole page showing self-expansiveness, which may be interpreted as the compensatory mechanism of a person who feels inadequate. Unusually large drawings indicate aggression or acting-out tendencies in the individual.

PENCIL PRESSURE

This indicates energy level. Heavy pressure indicates a high energy level, tension, anxiety and an approach to life that is assertive as well as forceful. In some cases it may also indicate stress and, in rare cases, paranoid tendencies. Low pencil pressure indicates low energy level, a hesitant personality, indecisiveness, fears and inhibitions and, in some cases, may also imply neurotic tendencies and depression.

DETAILING

Normal individuals include essential details in their drawings. In a DAP, the essential details include a head, trunk, two legs, two arms, eyes, a nose, mouth and two ears (unless the omission is accounted for by the mode of presentation, say, a profile of a person). When any of these details is missing from the drawing of a normal adult with average intelligence, it suggests intellectual deterioration or serious behavioral disorder. Lack of details suggests possible withdrawal, depression whereas excessive detailing may suggest obsessive-compulsive tendencies, rigidity or anxiety.

PLACEMENT OF THE DRAWING

When the subject draws in the middle of the page it implies normalcy. Placement onto the right side of the page is indicative of stability, controlled behavior, as well as a willingness to postpone gratification. When the drawing is placed on the left side it means impulsiveness, acting-out behavior and a tendency towards immediate emotional satisfaction. Drawings placed on the upper part of the page imply a high drive level, great striving for achievement, striving for difficult goals with a great determination to attain them. It may also indicate the stress encountered by the patient due to his high aspirations.

Drawings placed too low on the page imply insecurity and inadequacy, as well as that the person is highly reality bound with defeatist tendencies and tends to concentrate on what he has at the present moment. Upper left-hand side corner may indicate regressive tendencies, withdrawal and anxiety. Upper right-hand side corner shows a desire to suppress the unpleasant past. The bottom edge of the page implies a need for support, high dependency, reassurance with a tendency to avoid new experiences.

ERASURE

The nature, type and amount of erasure committed in a drawing speaks a great deal about an individual's personality. Excessive erasures show uncertainty, conflict, restlessness, and indecisiveness.

When repeated attempts at producing a drawing better than the previous one fail despite erasures and redrawing, it indicates a high degree of anxiety and conflict. If the head is drawn and redrawn, the problem tends to lie in the head, that is, it is psychological, emotional or related to intellect. If any other body part is drawn and redrawn, it implies somatization. In addition, excessive shading implies an agitated mental state and a messy drawing means that conflicts are causing anxiety.

In addition to these broad indicators, the analysis of the content of drawings provides insight into the individual's difficulties and conflicts. Given next are a few of the content interpretation categories and what they imply in terms of personality and emotions etc.

HEAD

The head is the symbol or seat of intellectual and emotional activity, fantasy and impulse. It is also a site for socialization and communication. Drawing an unusually large head means an inflated ego, overvaluation of intellectual capacity, high achievement orientation and high fantasy. On the other hand, drawing an unusually small head suggests inadequate intellect and feelings of helplessness. Overemphasis of hair on head, chest implies virility, striving, sexual pre-occupation and compensation for sexual inadequacy, anger, aggressive tendencies and narcissism.

FACIAL FEATURES

Facial features are a major source of sensory satisfaction or dissatisfaction, as well as the seat of interpersonal communication. A drawing in which facial features are totally omitted imply the possibility of psychosis, evasiveness and superficial interpersonal relationships and a certain degree of withdrawal from the environment and from others. Large eyes imply suspicion paranoia, and hypersensitivity to social opinions. Drawings with small, closed eyes imply introversion, self-absorbing tendencies, schizoid personality, and communication difficulties.

NOSE

The nose is the symbol of power motive; a phallic symbol. The larger the nose, the greater the need to dominate, the more egoistic the individual. A small nose implies insecurity, submissiveness, and inadequacy. When the nose is omitted altogether it implies a shy, withdrawn, depressive personality style. If an adult draws a nose like ▲ (triangle) or ● (button) it shows a high degree of immaturity. A strongly pointed nose suggests acting-out tendencies.

MOUTH

When a person has problems in drawing the mouth, it could indicate speech problems or eating problems. If the mouth is emphasized, there could be a dependency problem, the person may be verbally aggressive and immature. If the mouth has teeth which are bared, it implies aggressiveness and even sadism. When mouth is omitted, it implies conflict regarding oral-aggressive tendencies, difficulty in communication and depressive tendencies. In certain cases, it may mean a highly withdrawn personal style.

EARS

The ear is one mode of being in touch with the environment. Drawings of a large ears mean hypersensitivity to criticism, ideas of reference, paranoid tendencies. If drawn by a schizophrenic patient it would mean auditory hallucination. If ears are omitted it implies, indifference (in a child who is less than 10 years old, they may simply be overlooked).

NECK

Neck is the link between intellectual and emotional aspects. It is indicative of the connection between ego control (head) and impulses (body). A large neck means a gruff, rigid, impulsive person who keeps his impulses from hindering his intellect. A long neck implies a tendency to separate intellect from emotion. It also means that the person is cultured, rigid, and overly moral.

When the neck is omitted, it implies impulsivity and poor adjustment whereas if the neck is shaded it implies emotional disturbance.

ARMS

Arms are important in interpersonal relations. Omission of arms implies guilt, depression, inadequacy, and dissatisfaction with the environment. Short arms imply passivity, fear of possible castration. Long arms imply extraversion, expansiveness. When hands are drawn outstretched it shows a person desirous of interpersonal contact, very affectionate and helpful. Large hands may indicate a desire to compensate for one's inadequacy. Small hands imply inadequacy. Hands with mittens mean a person who is reserved or has aggressive tendencies. Clenched fingers mean anger and rebellion.

To sum up, in DAP the indicators of psychopathology include gross asymmetry, omission of neck and a figure larger than nine inches as seen in impulsivity. Insecurity, inadequacy and shyness in a person are evident from slanting figures, tiny heads, omission of mouth, nose, hands, arms, legs or feet, short arms, and disproportionately big or small figures. Signs of anxiety can be inferred from shading of the face, and body, legs pressed together and omission of eyes. In spite of the clinician's instructions to draw a person, the drawing may include a cloud, flying birds, rain etc. Anger/aggression are indicated by crossed eyes, or triangles for eyes, presence of teeth, long arms (bigger than the head) and nude figures. Indicators of emotional distress or disorders may be obtained when the following are a part of the drawing— poor integration of parts of figures, shading of the face or any body part, tiny figures (less than two inches), transparent figures (drawing the insides of the body implies poor reality testing and psychotic tendencies), body parts cut off, monstrous or grotesque figures and three or more figures spontaneously drawn.

In addition to DAP, clinicians may ask the patient to draw a house and tree. Together, all these can yield rich information about the inner dynamics of a person. The House–Tree–Person drawing process stimulates free and open verbalization, and since they are familiar objects, both children and adults are willing to draw them. Some of the important aspects of house and tree drawings have been discussed briefly next.

Drawings of houses

The house is a symbolic representation of the self and of basic childhood and adulthood experiences. House drawings reflect the individual home-life and the quality of his relationship with his family. Sometimes they may be indicative of a person's past house or one which he aspires for, or a combination of both. *Size:* A very small house would suggest withdrawal tendencies, feelings of inadequacy, possibly neurotic whereas a very large house suggests feelings of great frustration by a restrictive environment, feelings of tension and irritability. Smoking chimneys are indicative of inner tension or anxiety in the home. *Walls:* are seen as representing ego-strength. Crumbling walls indicate that the person is making an extreme effort to maintain ego intactness, weak or faint wall lines imply feelings of tension or weak ego. *Doors:* The manner in which the door is drawn is indicative of the patient's contact with the environment. Absence of doors suggests inaccessibility and withdrawal tendencies, feelings of isolation, feelings of social inadequacy and indecision are suggested by very small doors. Very large doors indicate overdependence and the need to impress with social accessibility. Open doors would imply a strong need for emotional warmth from the environment. Doors with stairs leading to them indicate that the person needs environmental contact but, at the same time, values his privacy. *Windows:* represent the manner in which the person making the drawing interacts with the environment. Those who draw locks on windows (or doors, for that matter) fear intrusion from outside and are guarded and suspicious. If windows are shuttered it implies withdrawal tendencies in a person whereas open windows mean invitation for open communication for others. *Perspective:* If the house is drawn with a bird's-eye view (that is with the viewer looking down) it may imply that the person rejects the home situation. When the house is drawn as if one were looking up at it, this is said to represent feelings of poor self or of rejection by family members. These people feel extremely inadequate and happiness at home is seen as unattainable.

According to Buck (1966), the inclusion of "irrelevant details", for example, grass, birds, sun, clouds imply mild basic insecurity, free floating anxiety and a need to structure the situation more securely. When shadows are cast by the house, anxiety may be inferred. Mountains in the background denote a need for independence. Trees spontaneously drawn around the house may suggest strong dependence needs. Inability to integrate the parts of a house on to a unified whole may suggest organicity.

Drawings of trees

In addition to drawings of persons and houses, trees may also provide clues to the patients' personality and needs. The tree drawing is representative of the self and taps deeper layers of the self than does the DAP. *Location on the page:* Placement on the left indicates impulsive behavior and that the person seeks immediate emotional satisfaction. Placement on the right shows is stability and a willingness to delay satisfaction. Drawings placed on the upper part of the page show a striving for unattainable goals and feeling of frustration, while a drawing placed on the bottom implies insecurity and timidity. Hammer (1955), indicates that a tree drawing in which the bottom edge of the paper becomes the groundline is a representation of an insecure patient who feels inadequate. Depressives too, may draw like this. *Roots:* symbolically represent personality stability. They may reflect feelings related to one's security motives and contacts with reality. Omission of roots implies feelings of insecurity and inadequacy, overemphasis on roots entering the ground suggest a strong, phenomenal need to maintain a grasp on reality. Shaded roots suggest anxiety and insecurity. *Trunk:* is representative of patients ego-strength, his feelings of power, emotional strength and adequacy. In this context, heavily reinforced tree trunks reflect the patient's need to maintain ego inactness whereas faint, sketchy lines used to draw trunks indicate feelings of impending emotional disintegration or loss of identity, along with acute anxiety. *Branch:*

depicts personality organization and ability to derive satisfaction from the environment. Fallen branches suggest the loss of the ability to cope with environmental pressures, while neglect of branches suggests lack of enjoyment in interpersonal relationships or dissatisfaction from mingling with others. Broken/cut off branches suggests feelings of trauma, castration and impotency and very faint branches suggest indecision and anxiety. *Fruit:* people who draw fruits on their tree drawings are said to desirous of nurturance. However, some clinicians are of the view that such people are capable of providing nurturance. *Leaves:* on the other hand indicate a desire for nurturance and dependency. Total absence of leaves or when foliage is omitted, implies inner bareness and lack of ego integration. Falling or fallen leaves show an inability to conform to social demands.

Trees casting shadows suggest conscious anxiety regarding past, interpersonal relationships that were unsatisfying. Psychologically disturbed people will draw dead trees and often such a tree drawing is associated with depression and guilt feelings, and feelings of severe inferiority. When a tree is drawn on an isolated hilltop, it may suggest feelings of grandiosity or superiority, even possible feelings of isolation and a struggle for autonomy.

word association test

This is the oldest personality test and was devised by Carl Jung for unraveling neurotic conflicts. The test is easy to administer and broadly indicates the problem areas. The reaction time of the response to each stimulus word is recorded and the conflict areas are inferred through the longer reaction time taken for particular stimulus words. Both, too short a reaction time and a delayed reaction time indicate anxiety. Responses of above thirty out of a hundred words clearly indicate a moderate to high degree of anxiety. WAT is a short test and easy to administer, particularly if the clinician needs quick indicators of what is causing anxiety. However, it should be remembered that WAT should be supplemented by other tests.

Sentence completion tests

This is another method of studying the personality, it is a semi-structured projective technique in which the subject has to finish a sentence where the first word or words are supplied. As with other projective devices, it is assumed that the subject reflects his own wishes, desires, fears, and attitudes in the sentences that he makes. Tendencies to block and to twist the stimulus words may be interpreted on the same lines as the Word Association Test. The test should be interpreted for clinical work from a common sense point of view or at a symbolic psychoanalytical level. Areas on which the test provides information includes family, social and sexual attitudes, general attitudes and character traits.

There are many methods by which the severity of anxiety disorders, consisting of phobias, obsessive-compulsive disorder, panic attacks etc., may be assessed. Of these, perhaps the most important technique is interviewing, as it helps provide the maximum needed information on the patient's condition at all levels viz., biological, psychological and sociocultural. In a few cases, while interviewing itself may suffice to arrive at a diagnosis and understand the underlying psychodynamics, in others psychological tests (paper pencil tests, or projective tests) may supplement and complement the information. Unless assessment is thoroughly and effectively handled, it is not be possible to plan an effective treatment program for helping the patient. Once the assessment strategies have been effectively used and a proper diagnosis reached, any one or a combination of treatment strategies may be chosen from the ones available for handling the problems of the patient. These are discussed in the next chapter.

4
Treatment of Anxiety Disorders

The primary aim of psychological treatment is to help patients overcome their symptoms and problems so that they can lead a mentally balanced and physically healthy life. In recent years, psychological interventions and therapies for mental disorders are more in demand compared to traditional therapies. This is partly because of their approach and partly because they tailor the treatment strategies to the individual patient's unique problems and needs.

Pathology is the result of a complex interaction of biological, psychological and environmental factors, and any therapy that attempts to reduce the symptoms of illness must deal with all three. Western models of psychological therapies emerged as a result of approaches that took into consideration body, mind and "subject–object" interaction. In recent years, however, the understanding of various mental health problems has become much more focussed and deals with cognitive, emotional, and behavioral issues. With the emergence of behavioral medicine, mental and even physical disorders are frequently handled through a holistic approach, helping patients adjust to physical, psychological as well as social areas of their life.

While many theoretical systems have contributed to psychological therapies, there has been an increasing tendency to combine different therapeutic approaches to suit the individual patient's needs. Such a combination of therapeutic approaches is called eclectic and the important prerequisites for such approaches include the following:

(1) Obtaining detailed information regarding the patient and his problems from multiple sources, for example, Case History, Mental Status Examination (MSE), interviews with the patient and his family, as well as psychological assessment.
(2) Formulating an etiological explanation after completion of a differential diagnosis. This includes the biological, psychological and sociocultural factors.
(3) Using treatment and management strategies that involve the patient, his family and his occupation.
(4) Adapting known therapeutic techniques to the unique symptomatology, and personal and situational demands of the patient and his needs.

The approach to psychological disorders has changed greatly over time, and the therapeutic orientations and techniques used are highly complex. The psychological treatment used can be broadly divided into four groups, viz., (a) relief of distress or maintenance functions (b) readjustment (c) restoration of functions in people who have developed a psychiatric disorder and (d) long-term reconstruction of patterns of thinking and behavior of the individual (cited in Gelder, Gath, Mayou and Cowen, *Concise Oxford Textbook of Psychiatry*, 1994, p. 353). While each of the above four treatment groups uses different techniques, all of them require that the patient and therapist be involved in a one-to-one relationship, and have a number of sessions varying from 4–5 to 18–20 or more, depending on the nature of the problem. In some instances, the patients are treated in groups.

Psychoanalysis

One of the major psychological treatment methods was psychoanalysis. This dates back to 1895, when Sigmund Freud gave up the practice of placing his patients in a hypnotic trance and instead simply urged them to tell him, uninhibitedly and freely, all they could about themselves. This, in turn, led to the development of the important technique of "free association", which attempts to bring into the conscious repressed material from the unconscious. One of the major goals of psychoanalytical therapy is to help the patient develop an insight into his behavior. It uses the technique of free association to make conscious the material which is unconscious, to deal with repression, to fill gaps in the patient's memory and to help the patient work through the painful thoughts and feelings she tries to keep outside of her awareness. Transference, dreams, resistance, clarification, and interpretation are some of the major tools used in psychoanalysis. However, this form of treatment cannot be used for any and every case and the contraindications include:

(1) Where there is an apparent absence of a moderately cooperative ego or when the patient is over 40 years of age, and lacks sufficient flexibility for personality changes.
(2) A mild neurotic disorder.
(3) A mild neurotic disorder which is urgent and cannot wait for transference neurosis to develop.
(4) A patient, whose life situation is unchangeable to the degree that successful analysis can result only in greater difficulties for him.
(5) The same analyst is already treating the friend or relative of a particular patient.

Since classical psychoanalysis was time consuming and no clear evidence was available as to whether the improvement obtained was due to psychoanalysis or first a natural remission, its efficacy was questioned. Further, a very long period of training was essential before a person could take up treatment of the patient. In addition, psychoanalysis was so expensive that a common person could not take advantage of the therapy. Thus, over a period of time, classical psychoanalysis became less popular with therapists. Alternative ways and means were sought to make psychoanalysis less time consuming less expensive, and requiring fewer years of training. Because of these efforts, many psychotherapies emerged of which some major ones are presented in the following section.

Psychoanalytical psychotherapy

As mentioned above, psychoanalytical psychotherapy emerged as a result of the problems faced in psychoanalysis. It required relatively less time, in addition to being more affordable by persons with limited financial resources. It took into consideration all the information obtained from the history of the patient's development, and his relationship with crucial figures during childhood and outlined a frame of reference to evaluate the patient's behavior. This form of treatment has been responsible for the emergence of various other psychotherapies such as brief psychotherapy, superficial psychotherapy, deep psychotherapy and intensive psychotherapy, all of which differ in detail but share a broad base of psychoanalytic principles and understanding. Some of these therapies are described next:

Brief psychotherapy

This takes less than six months, covers a course of six interviews and requires a good working format. In this 15–20 minutes constitute a session instead of one hour as in psychoanalytical psychotherapy.

Superficial psychotherapy

This attempts only a superficial understanding of the patient, does not deal with unconscious material, and has modest and limited goals of treatment.

Intensive psychotherapy

This deals with unconscious material and aims at personality changes. Each of these therapies may use techniques of psychoanalysis including free-association, transference etc. However, depending on the emphasis given by the therapist on free association, these therapies may be directive (uses less free association) or non-directive (uses more free association).

Insight therapy

This is based essentially on psychoanalytic understanding (*Stewart* and *Levin, 1967,* in *Friedman, Kaplan and Kaplan*, p. 1209). The emphasis in this form of therapy is to help the patient gain new insight into the dynamics of her feelings, responses and behaviors, primarily with respect to her current relations with other individuals. The insights may be emotional, ostensive, intellectual, or nominal. Insight therapy is the treatment of choice for a patient who has a fairly adequate ego strength to bear on his problems, but who, for some reason, cannot undergo analysis (*Stewart* and *Levin, 1967,* in *Friedman, Kaplan and Kaplan*, p. 1212). The effectiveness of this therapy is measured by the extent to which the patient obtains progressive freedom from unrealistic inhibitions, develops secure inner controls over impulsive behavior, and feels confident about his ability to deal with problems related herself and others.

Supportive psychotherapy

In this therapy, greater emphasis is placed on support than on other processes. While all psychotherapies may have elements of insight, support and relationship, they differ mainly in the relative emphasis and priority the therapist gives to each element. The goal of this therapy is limited and offers support to the person concerned during a period of disability, illness, turmoil or temporary decompensation. Supportive psychotherapy, which is given by an authority figure (expert), helps a patient tide over short episodes of illness or personal distress that cannot be resolved completely. The aim is to reduce distress, not to bring about any core change in personality. This kind of therapy relies on warmth, friendliness and strong leadership qualities. Support is given in the development of legitimate independence, and in pleasurable and non-destructive sublimation. In addition, guidance and advice is provided on current problems and issues. Here, the verbalization of unexpressed, strong emotions brings considerable relief to the patient, leading to a reduction of tension and anxiety. Supportive psychotherapy, if rightly used, is of great value and is a rewarding experience for therapists.

Relationship therapy

This therapy aims restoring the status quo ante, changing personality patterns and decreasing the patient's vulnerability to external pressures. It depends on a relationship between the patient and therapist without a sense of conscious effort. It uses support as the main method, in addition to establishing reliable, helpful relationship the patient can experience mature growth in his own self. The therapist maintains a productive psychotherapeutic approach and "rears" rather than "treats" the patient. Thus, there is a defined, limited, and corrective emotional experience.

Counseling

Counseling is an important technique in helping patients deal with stressful problems and making changes in their lives. It is used in a variety of problems and its basic techniques are similar to those of supportive psychotherapy. In addition, it uses techniques that can bring about a change in the lifestyle and adjustment ability of the person.

Behavior therapy

This technique is a relatively recent development in the field of psychotherapy. It constitutes an attempt to alleviate problems by controlling the learning behavior of the patient and is based on three principles of controlling and modifying behavior, namely:

(1) Behavior that occurs in a particular situation can be changed or modified.
(2) Change in the antecedent situational events can bring about change from maladaptive to adaptive behavior.
(3) Altering the situational consequence to the behavior can influence future behavior.

Behavior Therapy is best described as an approach rather than a specific treatment technique. It is derived from principles of learning and believes that all behaviors are learned and hence can be unlearned. The goal of behavior therapy in problem solving follows a typical course: determining the behavior to be modified, establishing conditions under which the particular behavior occurs, identifying factors that make the behavior persist, selecting a set of treatment conditions, and arranging a schedule for re-training.

Among the various techniques used in behavior therapy are relaxation training, graduated exposure technique, self control training, systematic desensitization, conditioned avoidance, reciprocal inhibition, positive and negative reinforcement, extinction techniques, negative practice techniques, assertion training, thought stopping and so on. Behavior therapy has been favored by practitioners because it is not time consuming and the changes which take place in the patient are observable and measurable. It offers a viable alternative to traditional psychotherapy on account of its greater effectiveness. More importantly, it provides for a person other than the therapist to be trained in conducting the sessions, thereby helping the patient to recover faster. Its greatest strength lies in its basic goal of establishing clinical techniques in the foundation of experimental method and procedures.

cognitive therapy

This is based on the premise that some symptoms and types of behavior are maintained due to maladaptive patterns of thinking.

The therapist, during sessions, asks questions that lead the patient to examine the basis of his maladaptive and illogical thinking, as well as the thoughts that precede symptom manifestation. The patient is stimulated to consider alternate ways of thinking about a situation and to test them to ascertain their applicability. He learns to recognize maladaptive thinking and to explore other ways of handling the problems and, by doing so, finds the symptoms reduced or vanish altogether. In certain cases, cognitive therapy may be used in combination with relaxation therapy to help the patient overcome the symptoms much faster than when any of these are used exclusively.

Group therapy

The main goal of this technique is to help individuals overcome their psychological, interpersonal and emotional difficulties. The various techniques used in this include psychodrama, re-education, experiential-existential techniques and group dynamic psychoanalytical therapy.

Psychodrama developed by J.L. Moreno (1945) is a form of group psychotherapy, which involves a structured, directed, and dramatized acting out of the patient's personal and emotional problems as well as his immediate group interaction. Forms of psychodrama have been used with children and adolescents, schizophrenics, neurotics showing poor motor pathology such as stuttering, tics etc., as well as with individuals who have marital and family problems.

Psychodrama is based on the principle that action and/or dramatic psychotherapy permits greater depth and breadth of awareness than is obtainable through verbal means. It includes procedures such as catharsis, abreaction, free association, acting out and specially planned and spontaneous encounters between persons. The major goal of psychodrama is not insight, but the promotion of spontaneity, perception of unhealthy responses, accurate understanding of reality and learning through experience. It is practiced in its original form as well as with variations, including role-play, leadership training and therapy groups. This method is very popular in problem solving.

Experiential-existential technique focusses on the immediate feeling of the patient rather than on the intellectual and rational explanation of an event. It is primarily a "here and now" technique, and emphasizes the group which serves as a setting for interpersonal and intrapersonal responses, referring as little as possible to the history of the patient. Acting is preferred to talking, feeling to thinking, and intuition to rationality and reason. In a number of cases, individual and group therapy are combined.

Family therapy

This deals with the patient's problem by involving the significant members of the family. It is based on the assumption that an individual's emotional difficulties stem from disturbances in the overall interaction within the families. It has evolved from the concept that there is a close interrelationship between the psychosocial functioning of the family as a group and the emotional adaptation of each of its members. Individual emotional difficulties are presumed to occur from disturbances in the interactions among family members. Generally, the first step in family therapy is to evaluate family interactions and the behavior of the individual members within it. This discloses any family pathology that may exist and may suggest psychiatric illness in one or more members.

Often, the family may be aware that there is something wrong within it but may not be able to identify the root cause or rectify the situation. The therapist initiates contact with the whole family in an unprejudiced manner without obtaining any history of difficulties and problems from the members. As the group tries to deal with immediate distress, the history of relevant and meaningful interaction in the present as well as the past clearly emerges. At this stage, spontaneous historical disclosures constitute a meaningful experience for the therapist who is able to identify the contemporary crises. As the therapist places this information as an active part of the present, the "live" past of the family, its interrelationships and individual dynamics become evident.

Family therapy is begun with face to face contact between the therapist and the family as a group. The manner in which the family members take their seats besides other members, the way they speak and smile, the tension, apprehension and frustration expressed either verbally or non-verbally give an idea to the therapist of the emotional climate within the family. It also provides clues to the confusion, fragmentation and distrust that exists in family relationships.

The family unit possesses a body, mind and spirit in addition to depth and surface expression, and an inner and outer face. As the session proceeds, the mask that each member wears is removed and the inner structures and conflicts are revealed. Family therapy emphasizes the principle of emotional contact in family processes and constructive results of fear, hostility and guilt. The therapist helps members cope with each other and facilitates the exchange of love and positive strength between them.

Though family therapy begins with superficial interpretation and intervention, it can attain greater depths. As the therapist stimulates interaction among family members and effects a meaningful interchange, s/he moves directly into family conflicts and engages in family interactional processes. Relatedness and health aspects are encouraged while alienation and sickness are counteracted. As conflicts emerge during therapeutic sessions, the defenses used by the family members are exposed and challenged. The therapist facilitates greater cooperation between the members in the shared search for solutions to their conflicts.

The informal atmosphere of the treatment setting and the therapist's efforts to inject some humor into the situation are effective means of piercing the pathogenic defenses. They also serve to ease the tension, increase participation and reduce resistance. The very presence of the therapist reassures the family members that they would not lose control over themselves.

The therapist provides them with elements of emotional imagery of themselves and others which had hitherto been absent. As new opportunities are provided to them, the family is able to test and retest its perceptions of self vis-a-vis its members as well as the whole. Family therapy aims to improve family "health" by removing barriers of isolation, aggression and guilt, and encourages mutual concern. With the therapist's help, each member attempts to express affection towards each other while becoming aware of feelings of love, affection and care within themselves. They discover a new sense of loyalty which helps them to identify and support each other. To sum up, the goals of treatment in family therapy include:

a) Resolving or reducing pathogenic anxiety in interpersonal relationships.
b) Enhancing the perception and fulfillment of each other's emotional needs.
c) Strengthening the immunity of the family against external and internal crises.
d) Promoting more appropriate relations between genders and generations.
e) Strengthening the capacity of individual members of the family to cope with the destructive forces from within and without the family.
f) Influencing family identity so that there is an orientation towards health and growth.

Family therapy is, in some ways, an educational process and the therapist serves as a symbol of the family helper. This type of therapy fosters understanding and resolves the conflicts and problems that led to the disorder as well as avoids secondary gain (a gain which the patient experiences as a direct consequence of the symptoms). It also facilitates reintegration of the patient within the family group.

Rational emotive therapy (RET)

This is a unique method in which the individual who feels inadequate and insecure and is bothered by irrational ideas, is helped to overcome them. The therapist helps the client give up irrational thinking. For example, if the patient thinks that he must constantly prove that he is thoroughly competent, adequate and an achiever, he is helped to give up this maladaptive thinking and do his best to be competent, adequate and achieving.

RET is based on the assumption that people tell themselves many impractical things, sometimes to the extent that their beliefs, attitudes and philosophies largely take the form of internalized self-talk. Consequently, one of the most powerful and elegant modalities that people can use to change themselves is to modify their self-defeating talk and sabotaging behavior. This involves seeing, understanding, disputing, altering and acting against their internal verbalizations. RET employs semantic methods that help in reducing emotional disturbances, and in changing thought patterns and emotive behaviors. If a person states that he "should work harder" or "should not hate my co-worker", he is asked to say "It would be better if I work harder at the office" or "It is preferable that I don't hate my co-worker", etc. In another instance, if he states that he cannot stop worrying, the therapist tries to help him change this to "I can stop worrying but so far I have not". When a person thinks of and declares someone a "rotten person", RET shows the person that the same thing could be stated differently, for instance "born and raised in a particular situation, the person is acting in such an unpleasant manner".

In RET, E = E' prime = E-e. Here, E' represents all the words of standard English and e represents all the forms of to be (is, was etc.). When a person uses E', the silly and unanswerable questions are eliminated and the person is able to expand his awareness of the environment. This helps identify ways and means to improve the conditions of the environment. When a person employs E' prime, the degree of completeness is eliminated. By sticking to E' prime and avoiding all forms of "to be", it is possible to get rid of absolutistic and self-fulfilling prophecies. Not only does RET emphasize human worth, but by helping persons differentiate between inappropriate and appropriate emotions, it helps them appreciate themselves better. RET makes a person observe his own feelings more fully and openly, acknowledge that they exist, accept their existence, determine their appropriateness and, eventually, choose to feel what he wants to feel. Some people do not realize that they act in self-defeating ways and do not accept themselves as being the cause of all their disturbances or that such disturbances originate in some of their irrational beliefs. Such individuals have to be helped to identify and remove their underlying, unrealistic ideas. It is not only important that they become aware of the misinformation and incorrect logic behind their ideas, but also substitute these with clear thinking, better logic and correct information.

Irrational and illogical ideas stand in the way of a person experiencing an anxiety-free life. These ideas are responsible for some persons showing a high degree of dependency, doing things to please others and constantly protecting themselves from outside criticism. Such persons do not feel satisfied and tend to blame themselves for things not moving the way they want them to. RET helps persons choose activities which they can take up and practice, and suggests methods to overcome their irrational beliefs and assumptions. In addition, it helps the person to recognize wrong thinking and perceptions within himself and correct them so that he can take up things that are of interest to him. The person is also helped to distinguish between blame and responsibility, and actual and seemingly wrong behaviors. He is taught that such behaviors do not solve any problems.

By helping individuals control their own destiny and conquer anxiety, RET helps them acquire self-discipline. It is important for persons, at the end of RET, to be able to feel how completely different they are at that point of time compared to the past. It helps them learn to accept reality and to strive for perfection, but to not feel bad if such perfection proves unattainable. In addition, RET also helps overcome the inertia caused by resistance. Over the course of the therapeutic sessions, the person gets creatively absorbed and learns to behave rationally in an irrational world.

To sum up, RET believes that irrational beliefs are major contributing factors to mental disorders, as they are evaluative and involve the dogmatic "musts", "shoulds", "go to", "have to", etc., which can all lead to evaluative derivatives such as "I am worthless...", and so on. Ellis described an A-B-C Model, where

A—represented an *activating* event
B—certain *beliefs* that the individual holds about the event and
C—emotional and behavioral *consequences*

The relationship is highlighted by A × B = C.

Thoughts or cognitive distortions are considered major features of distress, distortions being derived from the "all or none" style of thinking which lead individuals to jump to erroneous conclusions. Such distortions also lead to fortune telling, negative focus and over generalization. In therapeutic sessions, the distortions are assessed and discussed, and patients are helped to work on their primary disturbance, after which secondary and tertiary disturbances are taken up. In the process, patients learn to recognize their cognitive distortions and challenge them.

Some of the techniques used in RET include bibliotherapy and bibliotraining, both of which help to get over cognitive distortion. In addition, faulty inferences are challenged, cognitive focussing is enhanced and patients are encouraged towards constructive self-talk and correction of misconceptions. RET facilitates patients to dispute irrational beliefs and spend their energies in problem solving.

In the treatment of anxiety disorders, the therapist may use any one or a combination of more than one of the treatment methods presented above. In the following section, therapeutic techniques for dealing with anxiety disorder are presented with case illustrations. For reasons of confidentiality, the patient's name, gender, occupation etc., have been changed so that at no point is privacy endangered.

Treatment of Anxiety Disorders

Treatment of generalized anxiety disorder with panic attacks

In this, the manifestation includes high, intense anxiety, accompanied by a large number of physiological and psychological symptoms.

Anita, a female patient, 18 years of age manifested the following symptoms:

chief complaints

Severe anxiety
Choking sensation

Difficulty in breathing
Shortness of breath
Palpitations
Headaches
Panic attacks lasting for 3–4 minutes during which she felt that she was "going to die" and that the "whole world is going to collapse".

When asked to describe her symptoms, she said: "I feel tense, I feel something awful is going to happen. I worry all the time, have palpitations, get dizzy and feel faint." The case history showed that the onset was sudden, the patient was normal and carrying on her work but suddenly developed these symptoms seven months earlier. The precipitating event appeared to be her visit to the dentist, which lasted for 5–10 minutes, after which she had these attacks. In the previous two months, these attacks became too frequent to allow her to carry out even her daily routine.

History

The first three sessions focussed on obtaining information on the problem, symptoms, the patient's interpersonal relationships at home and outside, her likes and dislikes, aspirations and achievements, frustrations and disappointments, as well as on the psychodynamics underlying the problem. It was found that from childhood, whenever she faced situations which demanded high quality work where there were high expectations of her, she experienced severe anxiety. The patient constantly tried to come up to others' expectations, especially those of her mother's, but often found that the tasks she undertook in order to meet those expectations were beyond her capability. This led to a feeling of helplessness and worthlessness. While pursuing her studies, for instance, she was forced to take typing lessons in which she had no interest whatsoever, and found herself not being able to cope with either her studies or the typing, and felt defeated. It was also revealed that her level of inspiration was unrealistic and this, combined with her failure to live up to others' expectations, made her feel disillusioned and unhappy.

The early sessions helped the patient verbalize her feelings and she was able to clearly express how her family placed very high emphasis on achievement, resulting in her feeling considerable stress. While she put in her best efforts, at the time of performance (such as examinations etc.), she always did poorly. She felt guilty and ashamed of her failure and was frustrated at her performance and so, in order to please her mother and others, she would agree to do things which she never liked or wanted. She struggled consistently to do things she did not want to, and her dislike and resistance deterred her from performing at even average levels. She managed in school in this manner and was eventually forced to take up a vocational training course (typing) she did not like. She did not have the courage to tell her family of her dislike and disinterest but joined the course to please them. The constant demand of family members that she excel at least in that, and her consistent failure to do well because of her inner dislike made her feel annoyed, dejected, unhappy, guilty, and ashamed. Whenever she had to appear for a test or examination, her anxiety increased manifold and she tended to forget even what she knew.

The patient was careful not to apportion any blame on her family members but blamed herself for her failure. As she continued with the typing course, she started developing a high degree of anxiety, palpitation, dizziness and so on which prevented her from regularly attending the classes.

The premorbid personality was one of a reserved, withdrawn, and anxious person who had very few friends. An accumulation of multiple stressful events caused anxiety which she tried to cope with by sheer submission to every demand, in the hope of being accepted by all around her. She felt very helpless and worthless that she could not assert herself and tell her parents that she wanted to give up the typing training. The visit to the dentist, much against her wishes, appeared to have been the last straw in a series of stressful events that sparked off the first episodic attack of anxiety.

The assessment was made based on the information obtained from interviews, case history, and mental status examination as well as the administering of psychological tests. Post-Graduate Institute—Health Questionnaire was used to rule out other neurotic disorders such as depression, hysteria and obsessive-compulsive disorder.

Differential diagnosis

The first step was to rule out that the severe anxiety was due to a psychotic disorder. Assessment clearly showed no psychotic symptoms or organic factors associated with anxiety, thereby ruling out psychotic and organic disorders. Secondly, it was necessary to find out if the panic attack was associated with a specific object or situation, with being alone or in a public place, both of which were found to be absent. The third step was to ascertain whether there had been any separation from attachment figures and since this was not present, separation anxiety disorder was ruled out. There were no symptoms of either obsession or compulsion. The symptoms of excessive anxiety and worry with the many physiological symptoms had, however, existed for more than six months (which were not specifically stressor related). Thus, the diagnosis made was of generalized anxiety disorder. Figure 4.1 presents the problem profile of Anita.

Analysis

The main intrapsychic conflict was that of hostility and resentment against those who made her do things that she did not want to, combined with the need for dependency, recognition, appreciation and support from others. The constant struggle to meet the needs of others by sacrificing her own, led to her real self getting lost and being replaced by an artificial self.

Treatment

The intervention strategies required a combination of supportive psychotherapy and behavior therapy. The patient was put through relaxation using Jacobson's Progressive Muscular Relaxation technique. She was instructed to maintain a record of the nature, type and intensity of anxiety the moment she experienced it. She

Figure 4.1: Problem profile of Anita

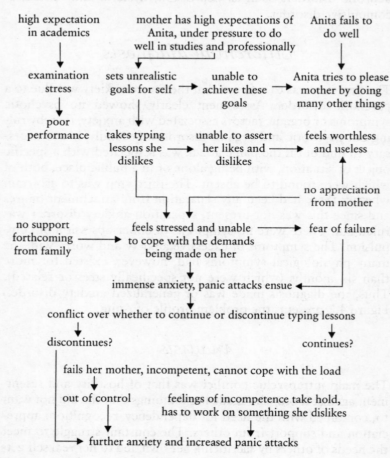

also had to note down what she was doing at the time, if any event took place then or just before, the significant person's behavior at that time, her action on feeling anxious, the consequences of her actions and whether others did anything to help and if so, how. These records were maintained daily and the patient learnt to observe her behavior at different times, before, during and after the anxiety and record her own and other's behaviors accurately. Discussions of this record with the patient revealed that whenever a situation demanded a certain standard performance from her, anxiety emerged. This became intense when she had to go for her typing classes or to the dentist. It was moderate to high when her mother asked her to do something which, again, required output of a certain standard.

The complexity of the anxiety causing various problems, their association with her past experiences, their effect on the present and future, as well as the relationship with the real and imagined events, were focussed upon and analyzed. Imagery training was used, along with relaxation therapy sessions. The patient was told to imagine herself in a situation where she experienced anxiety and was immediately put through relaxation, which reduced or removed the anxiety. Once the patient was able to understand some of the dynamics of her conflict, she was given training in self-assertion to enable her to verbalize her feelings of dissatisfaction and state what she wanted for herself. She was made to learn how to use a "problem focussed" strategy instead of an "emotion focussed" strategy for coping with stress.

Supportive therapy was taken up to make the patient feel comfortable with her own potentialities and capabilities. Relieving her of the guilt consequent to her failure to reach the standards set by her parents was an important focus of the supportive therapy. While relaxing, the patient learned to accept herself and her abilities in as realistic a manner as possible. She was helped to discuss her positive than negative qualities, and how she could use them to focus on her assets and strengths rather than on her liabilities. In the supportive therapy sessions, the patient was encouraged to set realistic goals and expectations for herself, goals which she could reach with confidence, bringing relief from her fear of failure and allowing her to act herself rather than as others expected. This made her concentrate less on pleasing others and start discussing her own interests, likes, dislikes and strengths. She uninhibitedly talked of her dislike for secretarial work and her desire to study more. She was helped in finding ways and means of accomplishing the goals she had set for herself. She also attempted to set a reachable goal and work towards it.

The parents were brought into the sessions, where they were made to understand the stress that the patient was experiencing and the role that they played in it. In the presence of the therapist, the patient was able to express her own needs to her parents without any inhibition and fear. The cooperation of her parents and their willingness to change, combined with the patient's new found ability to express herself before her parents without fear, brought about a change in their interactions.

While the sessions continued, the patient carried on with her daily record. Her maladaptive ways of thinking were identified and understood with their help. She was asked questions that led her to examine the illogical basis of her thinking, as for example, during her intense anxiety "everything will collapse", she was asked to consider why such a thing had not occurred during the anxiety episode. She was encouraged to consider alternate ways of looking at problems, instead of always from a negative angle. For example, she was asked to think of her fear of "everything collapsing" (which made her anxious) as being a consequence of heightened anxiety and not of any breakdown. She was encouraged to test these alternate explanations by diverting her attention from thoughts of disaster to something more pleasant and seeing if her palpitations reduced.

Thus, this treatment focussed on (a) exposure to anxiety provoking situations (b) various methods which could be employed to overcome anxiety, especially relaxation imagery training and cognitive therapy and (c) supportive therapy.

Treatment of Phobic Disorder

In phobic disorder, as in Generalized Anxiety Disorder, there is a high degree of anxiety in the patient. Here, the avoidance of situations that provoke anxiety as well as anticipatory anxiety are likely to be encountered. Anxiety provoking situations might be natural phenomena (such as lightning, thunder) or living creatures (insects, dogs) or specific situations (closed space, crowded areas).

In clinical settings, three groups of phobic disorders are recognized namely, simple, social, and agoraphobia. In simple phobia, the patient is inappropriately anxious in the presence of a particular object or situation and avoids it. The patient may show psychological and physical symptoms of anxiety pertaining to the gastro-intestinal or cardiovascular systems, or sleep disturbances etc.

Simple phobia is classified by the name of the anxiety causing stimulus, such as acrophobia (fear of heights), claustrophobia (closed spaces), and zoophobia (animals). Most of these begin in childhood and disappear as the child grows up. These phobias may be described as conditioned fear responses to a very frightening experience. If they continue beyond childhood, they take the shape of simple phobias.

In *agoraphobia*, patients show extreme anxiety when they are away from home, in crowds or in situations where they cannot leave easily. The symptoms are similar to generalized anxiety disorder, with depression and depersonalization occurring in a few cases. Broadly, the agoraphobic symptoms can be grouped under panic attacks and anxious thoughts. Many situations—such as being in cinema halls or travelling in public transport—can provoke anxiety and tension, and anticipatory anxiety is common in the sense that the mere idea of travelling in a public transport or going to a certain place gives rise to it. In other cases, the patient may encounter obsessional symptoms and depersonalization as well. It has been noted that an initial, spontaneous panic attack followed by avoidance behavior helps reduce anxiety which, in turn, helps maintain symptoms. A case illustration shows how a patient with phobic disorder was helped.

A 32-year old homemaker, Mrs Rani Devi with two children (aged six and four), manifested the following symptoms:

chief complaints

Extreme anxiety
Panic attacks when travelling
Palpitations, sweating, cold extremities during panic attack
Choking sensation and a strong drive to get out of the transport and run
Extreme apprehension that something terrible would happen if she did not get out

Inability to sleep, depression, shame and misery about her panic attacks and irrational fears

When asked to describe she stated that she could not travel alone in any public transport irrespective of the distance involved, and when she did try to travel she ended up with severe panic attacks, leading her to abandon the journey. In recent times, the panic attacks forced her to stay back home. She kept worrying about these attacks and so could not do even her household work properly. If at all she had to go out, she walked the entire distance rather than travel by any public transport. Earlier, she was able to travel if accompanied by her husband but now she was not able to do so.

History

Detailed history revealed that the attack was sudden and could not be related to any initiating or maintaining event or situation. From childhood she had been a shy and timid person who clung to her mother constantly. As a child she had been rather insecure, in contrast to her brother and elder sister who were bright, confident and secure. Both were married, had their own families, and visited the patient's family occasionally.

She was born 8 years after her elder sister and the parents hoped for a second son but it was not to be, and the mother was disappointed at the newborn child being a girl. Being sick herself and not feeling like taking up the responsibility of bringing up this child, she sent her to her sister's place where she was not very welcome. The patient always wished to go back to her parents but this was possible only when she was around 11 years of age. She was always angry with her mother for sending her away from home and often thought that her mother deserved to be sick as she had rejected her. Such thoughts used to make her feel guilty and ashamed and, in those days, she used to get rid of these feelings by tapping thrice on a table or wearing a particular dress, etc. Such behavior disappeared on its own, and after marriage, everything appeared to be fine.

Her hostility towards her mother, however, continued although it never got expressed in any outward form. After marriage, she settled down in Delhi. Her relatives expected her to visit them and when she did, they had much advice to give especially asking her to visit her mother. There was too much interference in her personal life. Her husband never stopped her from visiting any-one. When she started staying near her mother's house, problems started arising as her mother expected her to visit her often and made her feel guilty when she did not. Many times the patient used to dream of her mother dead or badly injured and in the morning used to feel sad and guilty and, as if to atone for the bad dreams, she made it a point to visit her mother, although with utmost reluctance. However much she tried, she could not get rid of her hostility, dislike and resentment against her mother. A be-havioral analysis of the problem clearly showed that it started with the patient experiencing slight apprehension when she had to go to meet one of her relatives. She sensed some kind of inex-plicable anxiety and fear but in the initial stages she ignored it and completed her visits to her relatives, friends and others. As time passed, she found it difficult to visit anyone except her mother. Even this she found uncomfortable and, more recently, whenever she planned to go to her mother's place unaccompanied, she found that on reaching the bus stop she experienced such severe palpitations that she was frightened and returned home.

From fears and anxiety that bothered her when she was travel-ling alone she found that, with the passage of time, she was not able to travel on public transport such as three-wheeler scooters and buses even when accompanied by her husband and children. She, her husband and children had planned a sightseeing tour but after going a certain distance she had to return due to severe panic attacks. These attacks surfaced all of a sudden, and although she was aware that her family was around her and that her fears were irrational, they remained intense until she returned home.

In addition to the panic attacks that restricted her outside movements, the patient reported that for most part of the day she also had several somatic symptoms such as feeling faint, severe palpitations, diarrhea and extreme nervousness. She dreaded having another attack and was extremely concerned about facing such a situation despite her husband's considerable reassurance, physical presence and constant support. At the time that she visited the clinic, she had stopped even making attempts to go out, and had confined herself to the house most of the time. She became depressed since she was unable to carry out even her normal day to day routine.

The premorbid personality was one of a shy, timid, anxious and sensitive person who succumbed easily to pressure, much against her wishes. The assessment, in addition to case history and MSE, used the PGI Health Questionnaire to rule out other neurotic disorders. The differential diagnosis was worked out as given in the next section.

Differential diagnosis

Since underlying depression and other symptoms may lead to a diagnosis of depression or anxiety disorder, it was necessary to show that the symptoms were flight symptoms associated with a fear-evoking stimulus (travel in public transport). It was found from the history and description of symptoms that panic attacks were spontaneous and not provoked by situations or objects. Since many physical illnesses and exogenous factors can cause the symptom of panic attacks organicity had to be ruled out. The patient was not found to suffer from any physical illness and no specific organic factors that could have caused the phobic attacks were identifiable. More importantly, the sudden panic that gripped her in public transport (three-wheeler scooters) and buses from which escape was difficult, caused her a high degree of embarrassment. She had no obsessions or obsessive intrusive thoughts, and so obsessional disorder was ruled out and a clear diagnosis of phobic disorder was made. The problem profile of Mrs Rani Devi is given in Figure 4.2.

Analysis

The main intrapsychic conflict was one of repressed hostility and anger at the mother, leading to guilt and shame in the patient for

Figure 4.2: Problem profile of Rani Devi

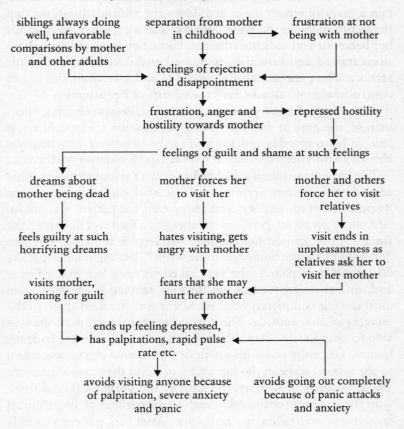

harboring such feelings towards a significant person in her life. Being highly sensitive with a strong superego, and faced with severe guilt and shame at her negative feelings towards her mother, and being afraid of hurting her, all appear to have led to a reaction formation resulting in phobic disorder.

Treatment

The onset was only for a few months prior to her therapy and hence it was decided that behavior modification could be used to help her overcome the symptoms. The patient was asked to maintain a diary in which she noted down the various situations that tended to increase the panic attacks. She was helped to monitor her behavior and indicate when and how her fears and apprehensions started and how they increased and developed into panic attacks. The patient was also asked to indicate what she did to control the panic attacks, and the results of her attempts.

After this preliminary session, which focussed on eliciting information, the patient was put through relaxation therapy. She was able to learn to relax quickly and in the next four sessions, was able to go into deep relaxation within 10–15 minutes of starting.

The patient was then asked to list down various situations that caused panic attacks in order of the least to most severe anxiety. By putting her into a deep relaxation state, the patient was gradually taken on to imagery, where she was asked to encounter the situation that caused her the least anxiety. In her case, this was "planning to leave home for some work". During imagery, if she felt anxious or panicy, she was asked to raise her index finger and, on her doing so, was put through relaxation all over again until she felt completely relaxed. She was then taken again to the imagery of that episode. These exercises continued until she was able to completely relax with the imagery of "planning to leave home". Once she was without anxiety at this level, she was taken to the second stage in the hierarchy of items that caused anxiety. The procedure of relaxing the patient and going back and forth with the imagery continued in such a manner that all hierarchical level items were taken up one by one. After this, patient was able to be totally without anxiety in regard to the anxiety-evoking situation in imagery. Finally, the imagery of getting into public transport was taken up.

During each of these sessions, in addition to behavior modification techniques, the patient was given supportive therapy. She was helped to understand how avoiding a situation helped her reduce the anxiety and how reduction in the anxiety made her continue with this avoidance. She was taught to break this cycle by just facing and encountering the situation first in imagery and later, in real-life situations. Many of her doubts were clarified and she was made to feel that there was someone to help her in case she had panic attacks while on public transport. By the 12th session, the patient was able to reach the level of attempting to leave the house with her husband and walk upto a point, every evening.

Her fear of leaving home reduced and she was able to do the relaxation exercises whenever she felt anxious or panicky. She succeeded in coming in a bus, along with her husband, to attend the therapeutic session at the clinic. However, there were three or four occasions when she went back home without getting onto the bus in spite of all the reassurances of her husband. The therapist took up these issues in her imagery sessions and the patient was encouraged to develop confidence, even when her husband could not accompany her. Although she was free of anxiety and panic when she traveled in imagery, in real life she was unable to travel without her husband, despite the fact that she had overcome her fear of travelling in a public transport to some extent. Around the 26th session, the patient was still not able to travel alone. At this point, the therapist changed the strategy and used flooding, that is, the therapist accompanied the patient up to the bus stop and traveled with her until the next stop. Then the therapist returned, instructing the patient to take another bus and come back on her own to the clinic bus stop, where the therapist waited for her. The patient was able to do so successfully, without any panic attacks. The therapist, for the next three sessions accompanied the patient, dropped her off and awaited her to return. After this, the therapist began to accompany the patient only up to the bus stop and the patient would board the bus alone, travel until the next stop and come back on her own.

During this period, relaxation, imagery, and individual psychotherapy continued. As the 40th session was completed, the patient was able to travel from home to the hospital unaccompanied. She was able to complete her household work, give her children company and became more cheerful as the fear of panic attack and the inability to stick to a routine diminished. At this point of time, a few sessions were taken by the therapist with the husband as to how he could provide patient with support without making her dependent on him. The cooperation of the husband helped a great deal in speeding up the patient's recovery process. After nearly 10 months of treatment, the patient was asymptomatic and the number of visits was reduced to as and when needed.

Follow up after a year showed that she maintained the improvement. The analysis of treatment shows that (*a*) The first issue to be tackled was the anxiety and tension in the patient and this was possible through relaxation procedure. (*b*) The patient needed to verbalize her fear, apprehensions and face the anxiety provoking situations squarely, which was done during the individual therapy and imagery. (*c*) The reduced level of anxiety and panic helped her to look at her problem in a slightly more objective manner. She was able to question her fears, monitor situations where she experienced anxiety, and reduce tension and anxiety by relaxation exercises. (*d*) Her realization that she, by herself, and by her own efforts could reduce anxiety gave her considerable confidence in overcoming the perceived insurmountability of an anxiety provoking stimulus. (*e*) The development of self-confidence, reassurance from her husband and exposure to the anxiety provoking situation with the ability to remain relaxed, helped her become asymptomatic.

Thus, in dealing with phobic disorder, apart from using the desensitization procedure "flooding" might also have to be used. Supportive psychotherapy and the involvement of a significant person in the patient's life can contribute towards a quick recovery.

Treatment of Obsessive-Compulsive Disorder

Obsessive-Compulsive Disorder (OCD) is an anxiety disorder where patients experience anxiety directly from a stimulus or if some of their behaviors (such as avoidant behavior, ritualistic behavior or thoughts) are interfered with. Obsessions are recurrent and persistent thoughts, ideas and images that are intrusive and unwanted; they are usually repugnant to the person, who attempts to suppress or ignore them because they invade the consciousness without his consent. A person suffering from this disorder is different from a psychotic in that he does not believe that his thoughts arise from an outside source or person as a psychotic does. Many symptoms obtained in obsessive-compulsive disorders are also found in generalized anxiety disorder, schizophrenia, phobia, depression etc., making diagnosis of OCD difficult. The most useful distinguishing characteristics of this disorder are repetitiveness and excessiveness of obsessive thoughts and behavior, accompanied by marked distress that interferes in the person's social and occupational functioning.

In obsessive-compulsive disorder, the patient may show irrational and excessive anxiety or worry, avoidance behavior not attributed to a psychotic disorder and without any involvement of organicity. He may have recurrent panic attacks, may be frightened of being in certain places and doing or not doing certain things. He has an excessive fear of a circumscribed stimulus other than the one related to social situations. The obsessions and compulsions cause the person embarrassment in social situations and, when accompanied by excessive shrinking from contact with people, lead to the patient avoiding the situation or engaging in certain ritualistic behaviors.

Another important characteristic of this disorder is the patient engaging in certain acts, or having unpalatable thoughts against his wishes. Despite his best effort to resist these, he ends up only with more such thoughts and ruminations. These obsessional thoughts are ideas, words and beliefs recognized by the patient as being ego-dystonic, which intrude in a compelling way in his thinking. The combination of being forced to have such thoughts and unsuccessfully trying to resist them, constitutes obsessive thinking. These thoughts, incidentally, are perceived as unpleasant, shocking and/or obscene. A case of obsessive-compulsive disorder, which was treated with an eclectic approach, is presented in the following section:

Mr Rajesh Raj is a 56-year-old male, married, with two grown up children (a boy and a girl), both well settled and well placed. He works in a flourishing business.

chief complaints

Intrusive negative thoughts ("son will die")
Intrusive aggressive thoughts about his daughter

Intrusive religious thoughts, abusive of God and religion
Indulges in compulsively breaking the idols of Gods, etc.
The patient was reportedly feeling blue, depressed, guilty, with
suicidal ideas and aggression towards himself
Insomnia, lack of appetite and lack of interest in everything
were other complaints

When asked for details, the patient said that it was extremely
painful for him to have these shameful thoughts involving his
children and God. However hard he tried, he found it difficult to
get rid of them. The more he tried to avoid these thoughts the
more forcefully they returned, making him feel all the more anxious and guilty. While at work, he found these thoughts bothering
him and adversely affecting his concentration. He had exhausted
all the leave to his credit and was on the verge of losing his job.

History

The detailed case history indicated that the onset of symptoms
was sometime in 1975, when he used to have repeated negative
thoughts with religious content. When the thoughts did not disappear he would clap his hands or bang his foot on the floor until
they did. He had been on medication for nearly 18 years and had
short periods of remission when the above symptoms were not
manifest. He was able to manage his work and routine quite to
his satisfaction. In the last few months, however, before he
sought help the symptoms had become exacerbated. Even when
he clapped his hands or banged his foot the intrusive thoughts
did not disappear, but continued to bother him. Most of his physical and psychological complaints had worsened, with the result
that he took long leave from work. The family history revealed
that his mother was a patient of OCD and that the patient, as a
child, used to be very anxious, a perfectionist and used to suffer
from severe anxiety attacks during examinations in school and
college.
The premorbid personality of the patient showed him to have
always been a highly sensitive person with perfectionist traits,

lack of confidence in himself and constantly worried about what people thought of him. Even petty issues made him feel guilty and unhappy. The precipitating factor for the present exacerbation of symptoms was reported to be the marriage of his daughter. He remained depressed in the office and was not able to work even at a minimal level. His superior, recognizing his illness, transferred him at his request to a department which had light work. The Medico-Psychological Health Questionnaire clearly indicated obsessive-compulsive disorder. TAT revealed intrapsychic conflicts regarding himself and authority figures in his life.

Differential diagnosis

OCD had to be differentiated diagnostically from generalized anxiety disorder, panic disorder, phobic disorder, as well as from depressive disorder. The assessment showed clearly that there were no auditory hallucinations and no symptoms of schizophrenia or any other psychotic disorder. There was no thought-affect-behavior incongruity or any type of mood swings. The anxiety was not of a free floating type, but was completely confined to the thoughts that intruded into the patient's thinking, thus ruling out generalized anxiety disorder. There were no symptoms of panic and so phobic disorder was ruled out. Patient was very depressed but did not show any symptoms of dysthymia or other mood disorder manifesting depression and related psychomotor retardation. Depression was directly related to his inability to stop the obnoxious and obscene thoughts that intruded into his thinking, and which he could not force out of his system. In the final analysis, it proved to be a case of obsessive-compulsive disorder (obsessive rumination). The problem profile of Mr Rajesh Raj is given in Figure 4.3.

Analysis

The patient had a highly punitive and restrictive superego, a weak ego, and a high degree of ambivalence. This could be observed in

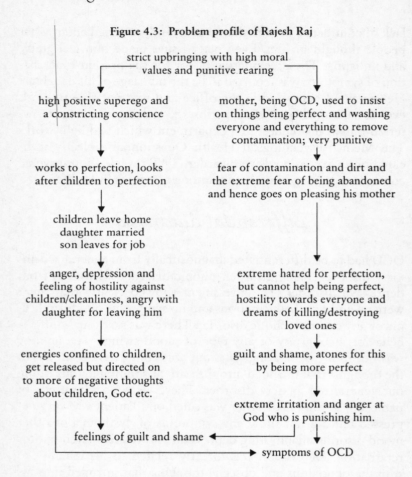

Figure 4.3: Problem profile of Rajesh Raj

strict upbringing with high moral
values and punitive rearing

high positive superego and
a constricting conscience

mother, being OCD, used to insist
on things being perfect and washing
everyone and everything to remove
contamination; very punitive

works to perfection, looks
after children to perfection

fear of contamination and dirt and
the extreme fear of being abandoned
and hence goes on pleasing his mother

children leave home
daughter married
son leaves for job

anger, depression and
feeling of hostility against
children/cleanliness, angry with
daughter for leaving him

extreme hatred for perfection,
but cannot help being perfect,
hostility towards everyone and
dreams of killing/destroying
loved ones

energies confined to children,
get released but directed on
to more of negative thoughts
about children, God etc.

guilt and shame, atones for this
by being more perfect

extreme irritation and anger at
God who is punishing him.

feelings of guilt and shame ◄—————

symptoms of OCD

his combined feelings of high dependency and extreme hostility
towards his mother which, incidentally, were generalized to other
female figures. He loved his daughter/son/mother and depended
on them a great deal for emotional sustenance, but also harbored
angry, hostile feelings towards them which manifested in dreams
in the form of his destroying them. In a mature person, love for a
person dominates over aggression—the latter playing only a
minor role. However, when regression occurs, there is a return
to earlier level of thinking, that is to an ambivalent mode. This
patient devoted all his time and energy to getting his son and

daughter well settled and had consciously only wished them well. He had a deep attachment to his daughter along with a lot of hostility, transferred to her from his past feelings for his own mother. When she got married and left home, he felt that she had abandoned him like his mother. OCD patients consciously experience love and hate towards the person (love object), thus, the obscene thoughts regarding daughter/son/God etc., appear to have obtained.

Treatment

After analysis of the case, a treatment plan was worked out and the goals of therapy were:

(1) To reduce the patients obsessional thoughts.
(2) To decrease his feelings of guilt, self-pity and worthlessness.

Treatment strategy included a combination of supportive therapy and behavior modification (thought stopping). While the former focussed on helping the patient verbalize his obsessive thoughts, soothe his extreme feelings of guilt, reduce his feelings of worthlessness and inability to stop the thoughts etc., the latter focussed on helping him use thought stopping and relaxation to reduce the intrusive thoughts. His attention was drawn to the good things that he had done for his family and the love and affection he had given and received from them.

His extreme attachment to his daughter and the pain of separation after her marriage were expressed by him and discussed at length. His inability to accept the separation and his anxiety at it were also dealt with in the therapeutic sessions. Since the patient was extremely anxious and tense, he was put on relaxation, initially using breathing exercises and then, progressively, muscular relaxation of the Jacobsen technique. He was told to do the relaxation exercises before he went to sleep at night, as well as whenever he felt anxious. During these relaxed states, the patient was helped to express his feelings regarding separation from his daughter, her future, and his dependency on her.

The patient prepared a list of intrusive thoughts that caused anxiety and rated them from the least to greatest. The therapist, after putting the patient into deep relaxation, took him through imagery where he was asked to visualize the least anxiety provoking thought. As and when he experienced anxiety he indicated it by raising his right index finger. On getting this signal, the therapist would loudly say "stop". The patient's intrusive thoughts thus ceased for a while. He was kept under relaxation all the time and then, as anxiety subsided, he was taken back to the same imagery and the process repeated. These exercises continued until the anxiety disappeared for the imagery of the intrusive thought. Once he was able to manage to stop that particular thought from intruding, he was taken to the imagery of the next item that is, the one that produced a greater amount of anxiety than the earlier one.

The thought-stopping sessions continued for each of the levels of anxiety mentioned in the hierarchical list, until the patient learned to remain relaxed and the intrusive thoughts disappeared. As he became increasingly familiar with the technique of thought stopping, he was made to try saying "stop" to himself whenever a negative thought intruded. Initially, the patient continued the thought-stopping exercises in the presence of therapist but later continued to do so at home and at his workplace. Gradually, the thoughts ceased to intrude.

In the psychotherapeutic sessions, the focus was on clarifying to him the shame, guilt, and feelings of worthlessness that he was experiencing. He was made to realize how his high dependency on his mother and female figures in his life, including his daughter, were reflective of his own feelings of insecurity. He was shown how, by depending on them, he tried to sustain himself which caused feelings of helplessness.

With the help of these sessions, the thought-stopping procedures and the relaxation exercises, the patient found that he was able to develop some control over himself and his thoughts. The self-monitoring exercises where he could observe his own feelings, fears and apprehensions developed in him the confidence that he could by his own efforts, effectively alter and control his thoughts from disturbing him. He developed an insight into the reasons for his harboring such negative thoughts. As the intrusive, obsessive thoughts gradually disappeared, he was able to return to work and effectively carry out his duties. This made him feel happy and comfortable, and removed his feelings of helplessness and worthlessness.

He was given clear instructions regarding certain exercises and assignments to carry out at home. One of these was going for evening walks with his wife, during which time he was able to share many of his thoughts and feelings. This helped soothe his tension. As the therapy proceeded and thought stopping was taken over by the patient, he obtained much needed strength and the confidence that his mind was under his control, and that he could lessen his tension, and stop his thoughts by his own efforts.

After a year's intervention (about 46 sessions), the patient became asymptomatic. The sessions were then gradually terminated. To conclude, this patient with obsessive-compulsive disorder was helped in the following manner:

(1) The first few sessions were spent in understanding the psychodynamics underlying the symptomatology.

(2) The patient's total lack of confidence, his high feelings of dependency and insecurity which were the root cause of anxiety were brought out in the open and he was helped to understand his anxiety in terms of these factors.

(3) Supportive psychotherapy was used to help the patient accept himself and his assets and liabilities with equanimity.

(4) Emphasis was given to his thinking more positively and focussing on his strength rather than on his worthlessness and liabilities.

(5) The use of the thought-stopping technique helped in immediately reducing his anxiety, which, in turn, helped to arrest the negative thinking.

(6) Self-monitoring and graded exposure to "anxiety provoking" stimuli helped in removing his unfounded fears.

(7) Clarification and development of insight helped him understand his obsessional thoughts and behaviors in terms of his very negative experiences in the past.

(8) The very fact of getting back to his work after a month of intervention helped a great deal in developing confidence within him.

Finally, his increasingly successful efforts in stopping his thoughts, complete elimination of anxiety, development of positive feelings about himself, interaction with his wife and sharing his problems with her helped him to become asymptomatic, which state he maintained even a year after, when a follow-up was undertaken.

Treatment of Social Anxiety or Social Phobia

Social phobia refers to inappropriate anxiety arising in response to a social situation, for example, at a party or in a restaurant where a person feels that he will be observed and criticized by others. This leads to an avoidance of such situations in part, or wholly. Patients suffering from social phobia experience anticipatory anxiety at the thought of even encountering such situations whether at parties, restaurants or meetings/sessions. Partial avoidance involves entering a social group but failing to interact, by sitting in an inconspicuous place. The symptoms of social phobia are the same as that of generalized anxiety disorder. While these patients have specific concerns that others will observe them critically, there is also a realization that such concern is irrational. Although the cause of social phobia is not very clear, symptoms begin in late adolescence. Social phobia should be distinguished from social inadequacy, where the patient shows lack of social skills, in turn causing anxiety.

Thus, social anxiety/social phobia is inappropriate anxiety occurring when a person feels that he is being observed and evaluated by others. The common theme includes being open to observation and evaluation by others, for example, while attending meetings, seminars, making presentations, reading, writing in front of others, eating in restaurants etc. These situations may be avoided partially or wholly and, in some cases, anticipatory anxiety at the thought of encountering similar situations may be present. Symptoms of social phobia are almost the same as obtained in general anxiety disorders. They range from physiological symptoms such as dry mouth, difficulty in swallowing, palpitation, difficulty in hearing, frequent or urgent micturition, headaches, tremors, and insomnia, to symptoms of depression. Psychological symptoms include irritability, restlessness, horrifying thoughts and poor concentration. Unable to control their anxiety, patients systematically start avoiding social situations though they would rather not do so. Psychotherapy helps a great deal as can be seen in the case presented here.

Nisha, an 18-year old female coming from a high socio-economic stratum and studying in a college reported the following:

chief complaints

Palpitation
Headaches
Confusion
Inability to concentrate
Irritability
Agitation
Tremors in hand while writing

When asked to describe her problem, Nisha stated that she was brought up in a strict, traditional value system. School life was totally uneventful and, for all practical purposes, could have been like that of all school-going children except for her not having any friends either at school or in her residential colony. Her best friend was her father who gave her the needed company at all levels namely, academics, sports and recreation. She jogged regularly with her father and always was a topper in school. Her father was also her tutor for almost all subjects, and they spent long hours together at work and recreation and, at times, even gossiped. The problem started a few months before she started coming for therapy. She got admission to an undergraduate degree course in a subject that she valued and was very happy. She loved going to college but somehow could not at all enjoy the gatherings, meetings, seminars, workshops and presentation of assignments, in all of which students were expected to participate regularly.

The first few months went without such activities as it was the start of academic session but, by the fourth month, group assignments were given and the patient was asked to make a presentation on behalf of the group. This was the precipating event as she was ready to do the assignment but not present it. She wanted the presentation to be done by someone else in the group but neither the teacher nor the group members agreed. Confronted with the choice of either presenting the assignment or obtaining poor marks, the patient became slightly anxious and developed the symptoms mentioned earlier.

The problem was circumscribed to the situation of presenting a paper before an audience, and caused high distress and anxiety to the patient. She clearly expressed that she did not want to present the paper before anyone as she was sure that she would "faint on the stage" while doing so. She had severe headache, could not sleep, and said she was not interested in continuing with college and so missed classes on a number of occasions. The teachers and her classmates, oblivious to her predicament, were determined to have her make the presentation. This was when she sought help.

The premorbid personality of the girl was a highly insecure, anxious, highly sensitive, intelligent, social, simple, passive aggressive one, with a withdrawing tendency. Sentence Completion Test was used to ascertain the nature of her intrapsychic and interpersonal relationships.

Differential diagnosis

Social phobia/social anxiety has to be differentially diagnosed from generalized anxiety disorders, depressive disorder and schizophrenia. Patients with social anxiety know that their ideas of being watched are wrong and they have a recognizable onset and shorter history. It has to be distinguished from social inadequacy which involves primarily a lack of social skills with secondary anxiety. This occurs in people with low intelligence and in a few shy people, whose social skills have not developed fully. In contrast, those with social anxiety have the basic skills but are unable to use them due to severe anxiety. In this case, social phobia was circumscribed to the particular situation of going onstage and to being evaluated by others. There were no hallucinations or delusions. Thus, the diagnosis was that of social phobia. The problem profile of Nisha is presented in Figure 4.4.

Figure 4.4: Problem profile of Nisha

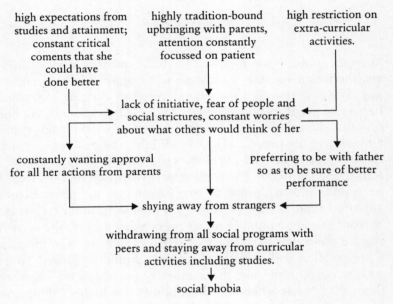

Analysis

The strong superego, restricted and isolated rearing, high traditional values and aiming at a completely perfect performance led the patient to depend on her father to guide and help her at all levels so that she never made mistakes. Even if she did, the father would help her out. There was a constant worry about her performance, not so much for herself as for her parents and outsiders. What she thought about herself had no relevance but what others thought of her and her performance was important. There was a constant attempt to play to the gallery so that others thought the best of her. Criticism by her parents made her feel that she could not be good and that others would laugh at her. Gradually, as she grew into an adult, these feelings became strengthened and she started avoiding all social situations. She felt that she was not good looking or well dressed and that others would never think positively of her.

Treatment

Since the problem was focussed and had overtones of social anxiety, the treatment strategy chosen was cognitive behavior therapy. The first few sessions were devoted to eliciting a detailed history of her fears and problems and understanding them. She said that she could not go on stage as people would laugh at her and criticize her presentation. She said that the manner in which she stood or spoke and the clothes she wore would come under scrutiny and criticism. She was extremely worried that she would be teased, and made fun of by everyone as she never before appeared alone in front of even a few people, let alone on a stage in front of a large number of her peers and teachers. She argued that for the course that she had taken, there was no need for such a presentation and that the assignment should be judged on its written content and not the manner of presentation. The very thought of "what others will think of me" was highly frightening to the patient.

The first step towards treating the problem of facing others and remaining in the public eye for fear of being negatively evaluated, was to ask the patient to maintain a diary of all the thoughts that preceded and accompanied the symptoms. She was asked a number of questions that led her to examine the logical basis of her maladaptive thinking. For example, when she said she would faint if she went on stage, she was asked how many people she had actually seen faint on stage. Of course, she couldn't name even one. When she was asked whether she had gone on stage in school she said had done so for a music competition but that then there were other girls with her and so the question of feeling faint never arose. She was then asked pointedly if that was not evidence against her statement "I will faint" and she replied in the affirmative. She was asked to consider social situations when she had not fainted and was once again asked that if she had never fainted in the past why she should do so now. Her maladaptive thoughts were questioned and she was repeatedly asked for evidence concerning such fears.

The next few therapeutic sessions directed the patient's attention to issues related to her fears in the presence of others. Since she was highly concerned about other people's evaluation of herself, she was drawn into a detailed discussion about the fear of evaluation itself. Four sessions were devoted to this aspect of her problem, especially what it was in the evaluation that caused her so much of anxiety and fear. She was made to write out and express these fears in clear terms to the therapist, who then put them back to her in question form. This helped her to face evaluation in a more realistic and objective manner. This process continued and the patient was soon able to not only consider the evaluation without heightened emotionality, but also to start thinking of alternative methods to counteract it. One of the self-suggestions that she was asked to use was "I have done my best and covered all points and have made sure that my clothes and work are fine. If people are still going to evaluate me negatively, I'm not bothered." Other thoughts included "I'll do my best and I am not going to worry about what the results are going to be" and "All along I have been worrying and found myself in a bad condition, why don't I try and do my best and not worry about the result." Finally, "I know it is my mind—I am capable of performing very well, what am I afraid of? I am not going to feel diffident and am going to be confident as I know what I am going to do." These thoughts helped her to counteract her fear of evaluation.

Two months later she had to give a presentation in front of her class; she prepared well and made the therapist listen to her presentation. The therapist appreciated her and asked her what she thought of her presentation. The patient said that she was satisfied and would do well in the presence of other girls. In the college, when her turn came for the presentation, she did very well and was thrilled when her teachers and classmates complimented her on her excellent performance. This reduced her anxiety considerably. Then came the annual day celebrations where too, she was successful. Over this period, she became asymptomatic with her anxiety disappearing. She followed the therapeutist's suggestion to go for jogging, play games with her friends and not confine herself to her father's company. She started enjoying the company of her friends and gradually began to spend more time with her peers, although she continued to depend on her father.

During this period, four sessions were taken with the parents regarding their daughter's problem. They were asked to spend more time among themselves and help their daughter spend more time with people of her own age. Their extreme concern and worry about her performance in examinations and their strong belief that their tutoring alone could get the best results from their daughter were discussed. It was pointed out to them that their girl was very capable and should be helped only when she wanted help and not as a routine. The parents were asked to look for activities for themselves, and let the girl develop her own identity. The parents, being deeply concerned about the recovery of their daughter, not only cooperated but also changed their lifestyle to accommodate the needs of their daughter. As the girl improved, they were even more encouraged to continue with their new lifestyle.

To summarize, it may be said that, to overcome social behavior, cognitive behavior therapy sessions with the patient and counseling sessions with her parents helped in getting the bright youngster to a normal level of functioning. Follow-up a year later indicated that the girl had maintained her improvement.

Treatment of Depressive Disorder

The central feature of depressive disorder is depressed mood, pessimistic thinking, lack of enjoyment, reduced energy and slowness. Depression is a common cause of distress as well as being a cause for slow recovery from physical illness. Depressive disorders are categorized as mild, moderate and severe. In depressive disorders of moderate severity, symptoms include low mood, lack of enjoyment, pessimistic thinking and reduced energy all of which lead to impaired efficiency. The mood of the patient is one of misery which does not improve, as would an ordinary feeling of sadness. The pessimistic thoughts are important symptoms, and may be concerned with the individuals' past experiences, or present and future concerns. The patient looks at everything pessimistically, experiences a total lack of confidence, and discounts his achievements and success as a chance happening. The future looks bleak and life not worth living. The pessimism is concerned with the past where everything s/he did was wrong and the calamities in the present are because of those wrongdoings. Most mildly depressed patients complain of low mood, lack of energy, lack of enjoyment and poor sleep and appetite. In some, anxiety phobias and obsessional symptoms, may also accompany depression.

Mild depressive disorder is also referred to as dysthymic disorder or dysthymia and the criteria to diagnose it include depressed mood and the presence of at least two of the following viz., poor appetite or overeating, insomnia or hypersomnia, fatigue, poor concentration and feelings of hopelessness. An absence of a manic or hypomanic episode has to be ruled out before making a diagnosis of dysthymia.

A mild depressive disorder can be very effectively treated through psychotherapy although, in a number of cases in the clinical setting, relaxation training and behavior modification techniques are also used. In the case presented next of a mild depressive disorder, psychotherapy has been shown to be effective in rendering the patient asymptomatic.

Rakesh, a young man of 24 years, unmarried, presented the following symptoms:

Chief complaints

Feeling sad, feeling blue, low mood
Lack of energy, interest and pleasure
Disturbed sleep
Palpitations
Poor appetite
High pessimism

Shortness of breath
Lack of concentration
Feelings of worthlessness and hopelessness

The patient revealed that the onset of symptoms happened two years ago, after which he had not been able to work, felt like crying most of the time, and did not feel like getting out of bed. He just lay down and did nothing the whole day. The symptoms varied in intensity at different times leaving him completely despondent, worthless and helpless. He had been on antidepressants and anxiolytic drugs for the last two years without much improvement in his condition.

The patient was also found to self-medicate and large doses of the drug had made him dependent on them, so that when he did not take the medicines his symptoms further worsened. The patient had finished school and when he came in for help, he was unemployed as he could not stick to any job. He also reported that his condition worsened before any examination/test or whenever he had to face a job interview or in any situation where he was expected to perform.

The patient was the only son of his parents and lived with them. He felt that they "did a lot" for him but he "was sick of them" as they had high expectations which he could not fulfill. He said that he felt guilty that he was unable to come up to even the minimal expectations of his parents and felt very unhappy at being unable to satisfy them in any way. He described himself as a "worthless and useless" son to his parents.

An interview with parents showed that the father was highly condescending, scornful and ridiculed the patient for being "nonproductive useless". Both the parents felt that they had given their son whatever was possible within their means, and that all they expected in return was that he studied well, graduated and got a steady job. He had, however, failed to do any of these and, when he had held a job in the past, he was unable to continue with it. The father pointed out that the son did not value his efforts to obtain a job for him. He just threw away the job, showing irresponsible behavior and causing worry to his old parents.

The father bemoaned his fate at having such a worthless son while other people had sons who were working, married and well settled. The mother had tears in her eyes as she also bemoaned her fate over her son. They both were unhappy that their son had to be brought to a psychiatrist for treatment. According to them, there could be no "greater shame" than this.

The premorbid personality of the patient was serious, morose, given to easy tears, total lack of confidence, timid and passive aggressive personality.

Differential diagnosis

The first step was to differentiate depression from apathy of schizophrenia. In this patient, there were no psychiatric symptoms of any kind, he was well oriented to reality, thought-affect-behavior congruity was intact. The depressive disorder was distinguished from normal sadness and depression in other psychiatric disorders. It was noted that the patient's depression was beyond normal sadness as it did not "lift off" after a short period with other distractions. Also, there was none of the typical sleep disturbance characteristics of severe depression disorders (early morning waking etc.) even though he reported having difficulty in falling asleep on certain days. There was no observable weight loss, or lack of appetite etc., which are characteristic features of severe and moderate depression disorders.

Depression was the first to appear followed by anxiety. The depressive symptoms were more severe than those of anxiety and this clearly pointed towards dysthymia. Psychomotor retardation due to substance abuse and organic causes was ruled out. Neurologically too, he had no symptoms to indicate the involvement of organicity. As the patient had no obsessional symptoms or phobic fears of any type, OCD and phobic disorder were ruled out. Dysthymia or mild depression was arrived at as the final diagnosis and a treatment plan consisting mainly of psychotherapy was worked out with the involvement of his parents. The problem profile of Rakesh Rao is presented in Figure 4.5.

Figure 4.5: Problem profile of Rakesh Rao

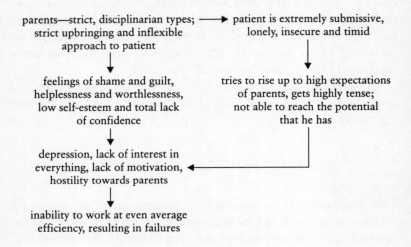

Analysis

The patient had no friends, only acquaintances, and he invariably confined himself to his room, lest his parents start preaching or pointing his worthlessness to him. He felt highly incompetent to do any task and gave up even before starting. He attributed his problems to the lack of support and guidance from his father, and added that his family environment, though not unpleasant, was negative and unsupportive. His father was not appreciative or encouraging of anything that he did and made him feel useless almost all the time. Any attempt on the patient's part to achieve anything was thwarted by his father's lack of confidence in him. In all, it was clear that the family was distressed and though they had love for each other, they made each other miserable by negative interaction. The result of this was an extremely tense atmosphere at home, which was compounded by the effect of the patient's successive failures, leading to depression.

Treatment

Before start of the sessions, the essential issues in the patient's life were worked out and the intrapsychic, interpersonal and socio-cultural aspects of his life clearly delineated. Analysis of the conflict underlying his pathological behavior showed that his non-cooperation was due to the hostile feelings towards his parents, particularly his father. These negative feelings towards the parents who were doing so much for him made him feel guilty and ashamed. He behaved in a manner so as to provoke his parents to use harsh words against him, (almost seeking punishment from them for his attitude).

The cause of his hostile feelings was the conflict between his own need for independence and doing something he wanted to, and the pressure from his parents to do what they wanted him to. He also had difficulty in freeing himself from his dependency on his parents, despite his strong desire to follow his own path. The parents' ambivalence was characterized by the absence of any loving support for their son, in spite of their extreme attachment to him. The patient hankered for something he was not able to get from his parents. The feelings of rejection that he thus experienced made him develop an oppositional tendency towards everything and anything around him. He constantly searched for something that he could do or achieve and feel satisfied with. It appeared as if he was trying to find a real self that had been submerged somewhere in the process of growing up.

In the early sessions of psychotherapy, verbalizing and abreaction were the main tools used. Focus was on the patient's experiences and feelings, and on allowing him to freely express himself. This cathartic process helped to reduce considerably the pain of rejection. In addition, during these sessions, the patient was helped in bringing out his negative and aggressive feelings towards his father without inhibition, guilt or shame. Expression of these negative feelings towards the most important of significant others in his life facilitated the emergence of a slightly more positive outlook, and made him examine more objectively the finer and positive aspects of his father.

Having reduced the feelings of shame, guilt and anxiety in the patient, it became possible to focus on issues related to lack of self-confidence. Since he felt that he was useless and incapable of doing anything, he was asked to list out five positive qualities in himself. With great effort he could write down only two positive qualities. The therapist instructed him to go home and think of the remaining three positive points. He was able to come prepared with them for the next session. The positive qualities he had included were that he was sincere, intelligent, a good person, serious, and one who did not hurt others. This was the starting point for the remaining sessions where each of these qualities was taken up and discussed in detail, with the patient giving examples from his own behavior, his interactions at home and in school life.

His intelligence and seriousness regarding studies were evident from the first division he had secured in the Class XII examination. He was, at this point, asked to indicate if this intelligence and ability to work could be transferred to the various tasks at hand. He said he could, but felt that he had lost touch with his work habits and thinking and was not in a position to "use his brains". He was then told to take up his positive qualities and dwell on them. He was asked that if given the chance, and if he was younger, how would he have used these qualities to approach a task. He said that he would look at the task, think about it logically and find a solution from the various alternatives available. From then onwards, he was given problems ranging from simple to complex levels to handle, and was able to give provide a number of alternatives to some of them. He was appreciated for this, which gave a boost to his sagging ego. He expressed relief that he could resolve these problems despite his "poor health."

From a state of total despondency, he came to view situations in a slightly more positive way. The problems that he solved gave him the confidence that he also could be an achiever. With support and encouragement from the therapist, he was able to realize how he could make use of his intelligence in a more effective way. This made him feel that he could consider taking up some course that would equip him for a job. Again, he was in a conflict about whether his parents would approve of a course that was not be up to their standards.

Here it was essential to bring the parents into the picture, hence family therapy was taken up with all three of them. The first three sessions were strained, with hostility surfacing every now and then, especially between father and son, and ended without any direction or specific decisions. Both the son and father clamped up when certain issues were brought up for discussion as each of them felt hurt by the other's remarks and no further conversation could be held between them. The therapist pointed out the need to listen to each other's point of view without getting upset since a different viewpoint did not mean an insult or rejection, but was just another mode that could possibly help in finding a solution to the problem.

The desire of the parents to see their son recover and work like any other young man eventually made them relent. They started listening without getting offended by their son's point of view. On his part, the son was able to understand his father's ideas about his future. In later sessions of family therapy, many issues were taken up by both father and son and discussed without much heat and emotion. The therapist helped them to see how the father could provide support to the son, help him to be independent and take up a job, as well as in working out the steps that they had to take to attain this goal.

After seven such sessions, all the three were able to discuss many issues at home without feeling apprehensive about who would insult whom. The father agreed to the son taking up a professional course, which could lead him to a good job. As the sessions continued, the patient's depression gradually lifted and many physiological symptoms were abated. A follow-up, nine months later showed that the patient was in the process of completing his vocational course, that he was cheerful and his home environment was more comfortable.

This case of mild depression was treated with psychotherapy and family therapy techniques. The processes involved were:

(1) Helping the patient verbalize his feelings without inhibition, thereby facilitating catharsis.
(2) Understanding of the psychodynamics and intra-psychic conflicts present in the patient and using them to help him

gain confidence, as well as develop insight into the "why" of his behaviors.

(3) Using exercises in problem solving and helping the patient take decisions on his own, thus enhancing his self-esteem and confidence and establishing faith in his own abilities.

(4) Using the attachment of the parents to the son and vice versa during family therapy to help make the parents understand the turmoil and conflict that the youngster was experiencing.

(5) A high degree of motivation on part of the parents helped in eliciting cooperation for the interactive sessions with their son in the presence of the therapist.

(6) The therapist, in turn, facilitated the restart of communications between the father and son leading to an understanding each other's perspective. This helped the son to see the genuine concern of his parents for his future, and for the parents to see how the harsh criticism meant for their son's good had unintentionally harmed him and brought about the neurotic breakdown.

Individual therapy and family therapy together helped in rendering the patient asymptomatic and brought him to a normal level of functioning.

An overview of the psychological treatments discussed in this chapter in reference to anxiety disorder cases clearly shows that there is no single, uniform therapeutic technique that is most appropriate. Instead, a combination of psychological interventions seem to be more effective. In addition, treatment interventions must be based on the accurate assessment of the various factors in the disorders and, more importantly, on the needs of the individual patient and his/her family. While medicines are a must in the beginning or when there is acute distress which adversely affects the patient's response to psychological treatment, most patients can become asymptomatic after psychological treatment.

5
Certain Problematic Issues in Assessment and Treatment

The two major psychological treatment techniques for anxiety disorders are psychotherapy and behavior therapy. These can be used either exclusively or in combination with other therapies such as family therapy and couple counseling, as has been demonstrated in the cases presented in the previous chapter. The need for individualizing the therapy to suit the patient's problem arises not only because each patient is unique, but also because his problem, personality, symptomatology, and reasons for seeking help are different. In quite a few cases, the patient expects an almost magical solution to his problem from the therapist. In particular, the Indian patient and his family invariably think that a pill, an injection, or at worst, an electric shock will solve the entire problem. These procedures normally being the ones they witness being carried out in hospitals. Thus, they approach a clinical psychologist or counselor with a similar orientation and when the therapist tries to talk about the patient's psychological problems and unravel the intrapsychic conflicts or interpersonal difficulties that have caused the symptoms, he meets with stiff resistance from the patient.

Since psychological treatment is essentially one of helping patients develop an insight into their problems and behaviors through the medium of the special relationship established by the therapist, considerable skill is required to carry on with therapeutic sessions. In order to be effective, the therapist has to be constantly perceptive and alert to the various problems and difficulties that arise in the sessions. Some of the more commonly faced difficulties have been presented in the following section.

Dropouts

A beginner therapist and trainee often face this problem. After conducting an interview for establishing rapport, the therapist may find that the patient does not keep his next appointment. This may be due to many factors including poor or no rapport, a poorly conducted session or one that ends up causing more negative than positive feelings in the patient. The psychologist conducting a session should follow the important principle of "start where the client is". In other words, starting with the patient's symptomatology and delving deep into those things that cause him the greatest concern. From here, by relating the symptoms to the various socio-demographic and interpersonal factors, educational and occupational areas, the information required for diagnosis may be obtained. As the therapist interviews the patient, he should get the feeling of having a pleasant conversation. Of course, the patient may be somewhat confused about why his family, educational or personal details are important and feel that the therapist should focus on the symptoms of his disorder. This is where the skilled therapist is able to help the patient understand how the problem is not so much a medical one, as psychological. He may give a simple explanation relating the "psyche" and "soma" in terms of a high fever causing depression, and a sad event diminishing appetite and sleep, which can help the patient understand the close connection between psychological and physical illnesses. If the therapist is able to convince the patient about the psychological aspects of illness, the first hurdle can be considered to have been overcome. One of the reasons for dropouts is the lack of understanding of this connection between physical and mental health.

Another reason for dropouts by patients in the beginning stages is lack of trust and confidence in the therapist. The first two sessions are extremely important not only for establishing rapport with the patient, but also for developing in him the confidence that by handling the psychological conflicts, the physical symptoms too can be effectively treated. The patient needs to understand that psychological conflicts can be addressed and dealt with only when he uninhibitedly expresses his core feelings. Effective, purposeful and empathic listening, combined with the assurance of confidentiality and expertise, helps in developing such a trust. Many a time the issues that the patient thinks are not important may actually be the ones that have to be focussed on by the therapist. The therapist must not only be well versed in the principles and techniques of interviewing but should also be alert to the various verbal and non-verbal behaviors of the patient, else the entire session descends into mere general talk leading the patient to dropout.

Yet, another reason for a patient to drop out of treatment is the feeling that he is not being listened to. While interviewing the patient or seeing him for the first time, it is important to talk to him first rather than to the significant others (friend, parent, spouse) who accompany him. When therapeutic sessions involve family members who are vocal and keen to communicate, a common mistake is to let them dominate while the patient, who should actually be encouraged to talk just witnesses the entire scene as a spectator and is reduced to a helpless, dependent status. Hence, irrespective of the condition of the patient, the therapist should make every attempt to find out the problems first from his point of view. This is all the more true for anxiety patients, who are already extremely anxious about their condition and tend to easily give up their rights and allow others to talk about their symptoms/problems, all of which only reduce their self esteem. Often, even if the patient wants to contradict what the family members state, he does not do so thinking that the therapist may not believe him or consider his statement unimportant. The therapist must ensure that every effort is made to talk first to the patient, either alone or in the presence of family members (if he chooses to), and give him the clear impression that he is the most important person and that his perception is important to the therapist. If this were ensured, the tendency for a patient to drop out from the sessions would be minimized.

Dealing with Negative Feelings and Emotions

Most patients try to hide important facts and negative feelings from the therapist lest an unfavorable impression is formed about them. Such apprehensions may be reduced if the therapist uses a non-judgmental approach and accepts the patient as he is with all his good and bad aspects. The therapist, for instance, can demonstrate to the patient that having negative feelings is as natural as having positive feelings and that the patient need not feel guilty or bad about them. A non-judgmental and accepting approach on the part of the therapist helps remove the guilt and inhibition patients often experience.

At times, a patient may express his anger, hostility and doubts to the therapist and show his familiarity with psychological treatments, saying that he would not benefit from them. Such doubts indicate that either the patient is testing the expertise of the therapist or has genuine difficulty in accepting the fact that he is suffering from a psychological rather than physical problem, one that requires psychological intervention. It is for the therapist to understand what the patient means when he makes such statements. It is advisable, in such cases, to put across clearly and in the simplest manner possible, what psychological assessment, testing and treatment involve, what constitutes the different forms of treatment (such as behavior therapy) and the reasons for using them. The patient may need an explanation as to why and how such therapies help and it is the responsibility of the therapist to clarify these issues in a manner understandable by the patient. Mishandling of the patient's doubts may result in him dropping out of the treatment program.

During sessions, the patient may show anger towards other medical/hospital personnel and may feel humiliated at being considered a "mental" patient. Even being sent to the psychiatric department is taken as an insult. However, if the therapist is a good listener who accepts these behaviors without any evaluation or judgement, the patient's anger may eventually cool down. At this point, the therapist has to soothe the patient's nerves and help him overcome the anger. He should set limits to the patient's behavior in the clinical setting.

When the therapeutic alliance, especially developed for psychological treatment, is strained or impaired, the signs must be recognized immediately and the therapist must make every effort to remove the ruptures and strains. The fact that the patient is at the receiving end and even expects "advice" from the "expert", does not give any "right" to the therapist/psychologist to give advice. The moment advice is offered, the patient invariably leaves the relationship. It must be kept in mind that although the patient may receive advice from many other people for solving his problems, in the therapeutic sessions it is the collaborative effort of the therapist and patient to find solutions. In other words, the patient and therapist work together towards a solution. The process requires the therapist to work with the patient to determine priorities, set goals, and maintain a therapeutic focus and structure, both within and across the sessions. Compromise on any of these core conditions may end up breaking the relationship and the patient dropping out. Difficulties also arise when a therapist takes up, or is expected to take up, the role of teacher, campaigner, bully or advisor.

counter-Transference

At times, the therapist may be unable to conceal his negative or positive feelings towards the patient, causing difficulties in his remaining an objective collaborator. Recognizing such feelings on his part as "counter-transference" towards the patient, the therapist should take the help of a senior colleague or supervisor to overcome them. To guard against such counter-transference, the therapist must check every now and then his own degree of involvement and engagement with the patient, especially how much he is identifying with the patient, how much he "feels" for the patient and how "hooked" has become in the interaction. He should keep in mind some of the indicators of counter-transference, for example,

(1) Telling the patient things like, "parents are like that, they cannot understand", "I also agree with you and what you did was absolutely right".

(2) Conveying to the patient feelings of sympathy and pity or getting angry with family members and showing his anger to them.

(3) Becoming speechless with rage and anger at what the patient has said.

(4) Getting attracted to the patient and giving him more time or sessions than are necessary.

(5) Going out of the way to help the patient.

(6) Feeling or saying that he is bored with the patient or does not like him and personalizing the comments of the patient.

Since counter-transference may also be caused by therapist's own personal limitations, his unresolved emotional difficulties and his unconscious conflicts, it is important to take the help of a senior professional or transfer the case to another therapist. Other important precautions to be kept in mind during therapy are mentioned in the following section.

Giving Advice and Offering Solutions

A therapist often finds it easy and comfortable to offer advice to the patient who, at times, specially asks for it. In the Indian setting, the patient looks to the therapist as a superior person in whose hands his future lies, and as someone who will guide him and solve his problems. It is extremely tempting for the therapist to guide, advise and solve the problems of the patient but it must, however, be remembered that such quick fix solutions to overcome the problem as perceived and conceived by the therapist are disastrous. No solution that comes from the therapist (and not from the patient) will ever be accepted, leave alone implemented. It is of utmost importance for the patient to perceive, understand, and visualize his problem and gain an insight into why he behaves the way he does. Unless he does so, no matter how convinced the therapist is about the right steps to be taken, no solution will be implemented. Even when advice is given where a patient very specifically asks for it, every effort should be made to see that the solution offered as advice emanates from the patient. This can be accomplished by asking the patient what he would do if a third person came and asked him that question. The therapist can then find out if the same advice would be applicable to the patient. From this point onwards, the therapist can discuss implementation of the solution, difficulties and how they may be overcome, alternatives that can be used by the patient and, finally, set the thinking process of the patient moving in a positive direction. Thus, however tempting and easy and less time consuming it may be to offer advice to the patient, it is important for the therapist to have complete self-control and desist from doing this.

Moralizing and Preaching

Lecturing, preaching and moralizing are a way of life with most adults, particularly when dealing with children. It is one of the prerogatives of older persons, who are expected to guide the younger ones; people in high positions consider it their moral duty to guide and advise persons younger or less experienced than them in the ways of the world. Leaders guide and advise their followers, trainers their trainees, elder siblings their younger ones, grandparents their children, who in turn do so to their children. However, all this moralizing and preaching does not always lead to a particular goal or give a workable direction. This is even more true in the case of patients. It must be remembered that a patient who comes to the therapist has already been preached, lectured, and moralized to by many before he is referred to the therapist. If the therapist also takes the same approach of "Do not do this..." "You ought to do this", "Don't you know that this is illegal", and so on, it only causes more pain to the patient. It must be kept in mind that, had it been possible for the patient to follow the earlier advice, there would have perhaps been no need for him to approach the therapist for help. Remaining neutral as well as objective, attempting to arrive at the basic cause of the problem and placing it within a clinical framework need to be taken up by the therapist.

Judging or Criticizing

A therapist should never judge or criticize a patient's response or behavior as this leads to withdrawal and the withholding of important feelings and information. For example, when a patient says that he takes leave without informing his superiors and if the therapist comments "how irresponsible you are", it would amount to the therapist being judgmental. If the therapist says that such leave taking indicates that he is inefficient or a poor performer it amounts to being critical. In the process the therapist may lose the patient.

Tackling Dead Ends in the Interview

As a therapist goes on with an interview or a particular session, he may find that he has come to a dead end. He may find that he has no more questions to ask of the client or even that whichever question he asks of the patient, he is back to where he started in and unable to proceed further. Such a situation is invariably found in a student trainee or intern and the reasons for such a situation could be (*i*) lack of adequate skills (*ii*) counter-transference (*iii*) total non-cooperation from the patient and (*iv*) limitations of the setting.

In the case of counter-transference, lack of adequate skills and techniques, or if the therapist is still on training, then his supervisor should be able to help him overcome the problem of a blind spot by drawing his attention to the problem in totality. The blind spot can also be overcome if the therapist points out a new direction to the patient. In addition, it may be worthwhile on the therapist's part to analyze his own questioning by listening to the interview on tape or reading the verbatim report so as to detect the area that brought about the stopper. Areas that need objective analysis to overcome the problem of a "dead end" include the interview session, questioning techniques, continuity and cogency between topics and bringing an issue into focus and moving from it in a meaningful manner.

Cases where patients become non-cooperative for inexplicable reasons need to be explored thoroughly. At times, non-cooperation is indicated by the total inability of the patient to convey or communicate any information to the therapist as well as by his giving a false impression or account of things being comfortable and moving in the expected direction. The therapist realizes that the patient is taking him for a ride and, under such circumstances, he may convey to the patient that there is no point in continuing the sessions. Alternatively, he could summarize what had gone on in the various sessions up to that time and indicate to the patient the possible causes of the problem and the solutions. As the progress made by the patient over the sessions become clear to him, he may give up being non-cooperative.

A blind spot may arise due to the setting itself. As for example, a setting deals with only certain types of cases and thus deals with all others in the same way. Some agencies may not be able to provide facilities to conduct particular services needed and hence one may be forced to a dead end.

Repressed Materials of the Unconscious

At times, unpleasant, shameful and painful experiences of the past are so repressed that the patient might not be able to remember or mention them. Whenever an event related to such an experience is brought to the session, the patient is unable to say anything and conversation comes to a total stop. The therapist should remain alert to causal antecedents of this type and, occasionally, repeat or put back questions to the patient such as "does this remind you of something that has happened in the past" to try and get the patient to talk about the repressed event.

Important clues to a repressed, past event are intrusive thoughts and images that recur in the course of a diary recording or when the patient is asked to jot them down. During the session, if the therapist notices signs of emotion such as a strained voice, sudden change in facial expression or tears, they should be noted and used for overcoming the blind spot.

When the patient tries to talk around an issue or shows apathy or a lack of emotional response to it, the therapist should be alerted towards a past repressed painful event and try to overcome the block. When a patient especially avoids talking about places/people on visiting them and refuses to discuss things associated with significant figures, it should be noted and efforts made to overcome this. Recurring dreams of the patients can also be used as a stimulus to help the patient freely discuss his problem.

Other problems that hamper the process of counseling include the inability of the patient to understand the rationale behind psychological interventions and treatment. In addition, it may not be clear to the patient as to what is required of him during the process of treatment. Problems in therapy also arise when the therapist fails to convey to the patient that the psychological treatment requires cooperation from him, and any reduction or removal of symptoms depends on the collaborative efforts of both the patient and the therapist.

Often, the process of counseling may be hampered if the therapist is not on the same wavelength as of the patient, for example, while communicating with the patient the therapist uses technical words, or explains the problem too simplistically. Problems may also arise if the patient shows a repeated lack of compliance with psychological treatment or intervention, such as not doing the psychological homework or assignment. This could happen due to: (a) insufficient preparation on the part of the client (b) the task may be too difficult or too much to handle and (c) the rationale behind the psychological assignment or exercises may not be meaningful to the patient.

There are many types of difficulties and problems that can emerge in psychological treatment. It is imperative that the therapist be able to recognize them when they occur and take adequate steps to deal with them as the success of the treatment depends on the identification and effective handling of the problem.

Appendix

Certain Common Techniques used in the Treatment of Anxiety Disorders

Behavioral Analysis

When a patient has been taken up for behavior therapy, the first step is behavioral analysis. This helps the therapist obtain a clear picture of the problems, causes, and the situations contributing to the problem, and plan therapeutic strategies that would help in overcoming the symptoms. This analysis includes:

(1) Details of the presenting problem
(2) Motivational analysis
(3) Developmental analysis
(4) Sociological analysis
(5) Behavioral change
(6) Analysis of self-control

These are discussed as follows:

Details of the presenting problem

This includes the nature of the problem, its behavioral consequences, its effect on the patient such as whether it leads to avoidance, escape or reassurance seeking. This procedure should also take detailed notes of (*a*) **behavioral excesses**—the frequency, duration, intensity and occurrence, (b) **behavioral deficits**—whether the behavior is sufficient in terms of the demands of the situation conceived, the frequency and intensity of the deficits and the form in which they occur, and (c) **behavioral assets**—the behaviors which are highly positive and which can be used for building up new behavior. In addition, this stage of analysis also includes the typical signs and symptoms, nature, precise feelings, thoughts evoked by the symptoms, and the degree of stress caused by them. An important aspect of this stage is obtaining a chronological history of all the important events that had taken place in the patient's life before the start of the presenting symptoms.

Behavioral analysis also requires determining the predictability of the problem, which involves frequency, duration, severity, and other situational factors associated with the symptoms. A thorough understanding of the impact of the problem on the life of the patient is to be gathered, along with the degree of impairment during work, social and leisure time etc., and how these, in turn, affect the patient and his family. Information is also obtained from the patient's significant others about the factors that maintain or exacerbate the problem, as well its effect on their lives.

Motivational analysis

Here, the main aim is to find the factors that motivate the person to behave in certain ways, and the incentives that are valuable to the patient and can be used in treatment—the therapist looks at whether such incentives have brought about any success for the patient in the direction desired by him/her. Motivational analysis also highlights the congruency and incongruency between what the patient says and does. It helps identify the people who have the greatest influence on the patient's correct and incorrect behaviors, and to find out to what extent the patient is able to relate incentives to his own behavior. Such analysis helps identify some of the major aversive stimuli that deter certain behaviors of the patient, both at the immediate and future levels.

Developmental analysis

This aims at ascertaining if the symptoms have, in any way, brought about changes in the patient since their onset. It covers:

a) The biological changes that occur as a result of the symptoms.
b) Limitations that have come about as a result of the symptoms.
c) Whether earlier treatments had any positive or negative effects on the patient.
d) The way in which the treatment helped in resolving the patient's problem.

Sociological analysis

This analysis includes the following:

a) The most characteristic features of the sociocultural milieu of the patient.
b) Whether the patient has noticed any changes in his milieu and if he can relate these to his symtomatology and behavior.
c) The patient's attitude towards the changes.
d) Any conflict in the value system of the patient and his early adult social environment.
e) Sociological factors that can be used to bring about a change during the treatment procedure.

In addition, the following points are also considered under sociological analysis:

a) The most important people in the patient's current environment.
b) The people who reinforce a behavior and/or who create problems for the patient.
c) The patient's expectations of the significant others in his life and their expectations of him.
d) The ways in which the significant others can be used in the treatment program.
e) All aspects of the support system available to the patient.

Sociological factors can be used to bring about a change during the treatment procedure. A typical social skill assessment technique is presented in the following box:

Obtaining a history of social functioning from the patient

Goal: to identify recurrent themes and problems.
Ask the following:

(1) The number of friends the patient had in childhood, adolescence and adulthood.
(2) The nature and closeness of such friendships.
(3) The patient's dating history, most notably the number, frequency, and success of romantic relationships.
(4) The patient's involvement in social clubs or activities.

B. Obtain a description of the kinds of social situations and relationships he or she finds difficult.

Goal: to specify difficult social situations.

(1) Be sure to cover the following situations if the patient does not specify them:

a) Work or school
b) Home
c) Public places (stores, buses, airplanes, etc.)
d) Recreational settings (parties, sports events, etc.)
e) Dating and sex-related situations

(2) For each situation described, ask the patient to describe how he or she interacts with the following people of the same and the opposite sex:

a) Friends
b) Bosses
c) Co-workers
d) Professionals (doctors, lawyers, etc.)
e) Service providers (sales people, restaurant staff, mail clerks, delivery persons, mechanics, property owners etc.)
f) Spouse, boyfriend or girlfriend
g) In-laws
h) Children
i) Neighbors

(3) For each situation identified in B (1 & 2) above, ask the patient:

a) To describe what happened the last time he was in that situation. What did the patient do or say? What did others say and do?
b) Determine what happened immediately before the situation occurred.
c) Determine what happened immediately afterward.
d) Explore the patient's motives in that particular situation. What was the patient's goal?

(box continued)

(box continued)

e) Ask the patient to rate his or her performance on a 0 (extremely poor) to 100 (extremely good) scale.

f) Ask the patient to describe what he or she may have done differently in that situation. If the patient has difficulty with this question, ask how he or she would imagine a person with no social problems would behave in such situations.

g) Ask the patient how often such situations arise in his or her daily life.

C. Ask the patient to rank the identified situations in terms of their difficulty.

Goal: to identify a starting points for assessment/treatment.

Source: Bellack, A.S. and Hersen, M., *Behavioral Assessment and Treatment of Anxiety Disorders*, Boston: Allyn & Bacon. Reprinted by Permission. 1998 (p. 237).

Behavioral change

This includes taking note of the following in the person's past and present behaviors:

a) The premorbid level (the patient's behaviors before the onset of the illness).

b) The events in the patient's life that lead to changes in behavior.

c) The level of change such as emergence of new behaviors, changes in the frequency of behavior and non occurrence of previous behaviors.

d) The conditions under which certain behaviors were noticed and if these have been transferred to other areas of functioning.

e) If these behavioral changes could be associated with the patient's interactions with certain significant persons.

Analysis of self-control

This includes ascertaining the following aspects:

a) The situations in which the patient can and cannot control his behavior, and that of others.

b) The negative consequences that follow such control and non-control.

c) The negative consequence of the control itself.
d) The situations and factors that help or hinder acquisition of self-control.
e) The conditions and persons who tend to affect the person's self-control.
f) That aspect of patient's self-control which can be used in the treatment program.

Relaxation Procedures

There are many relaxation procedures, e.g., Jacobsons Progressive Muscular Relaxation, Autogenic Training, Shavasana, Yoganidra, Transcendental Meditation and Hypnotic Relaxation. Relaxation is an antidote to stress and helps establish homeostasis between the sympathetic and parasympathetic systems, and strengthens discrimination through positive psychosomatic currents. The most commonly used method of relaxation is that of Jacobson's Progressive Muscular Relaxation. The basic steps have been listed in the following section. Before starting relaxation, the following aspects have to be borne in mind:

The room/the setting

The relaxation room should be:

- Dimly lit
- Partly soundproof
- Comfortable, with a couch and coir mattress of one-inch thickness; no pillows to be used

The patient

After being welcomed and made comfortable must be instructed to:

- Lie down in a supine position
- Loosen hair if tied up in a bun
- Remove watch, shoes and other tightly worn accessories

Discussion with the patient

- The patient's life-style, to ascertain whether it is conducive to relaxation.
- Intake of tea, coffee or any stimulants by the patient which, in the opinion of the therapist, needs be reduced.
- The patient's occupation, leisure activities and sleep patterns.
- Help the patient identify and spend time in relaxing activities.
- Give the patient a feeling that it is possible for the patient and anyone who wants, to develop the ability, to relax through regular practice.
- Help the patient to carry on all activities in a relaxed manner.
- Help the patient systematically record in a diary the different times when tension is built up.
- Help patient to obtain information as to when to anticipate tension and relax at the earliest signs.

Instructions for relaxation

- The therapist should give the instructions in a relaxed, soothing voice and should combine elements of focussing on actual bodily sensations, warmth and relaxation experience.
- Give instructions for breathing so that the patient is made aware of his own breathing.
- Give instructions for mental relaxation in which the patient is able to have an imagery of relaxing scenes, the details of which are suggested by the therapist.
- The procedure of relaxation begins from relaxing of the head muscle groups, progresses on to the muscle group of neck, shoulders, arms, chest and lungs, the back, the stomach, hip, legs and feet.
- Separately tense and relax the individual muscle groups with all groups covered in this manner. It must be remembered that all muscle groups need to be *tensed* and *relaxed twice*.
- The tension should be held on for about 5 seconds.
- Releasing of the tension should be slow, and at the same time, the patient should be told to silently tell himself "relax and let go".
- Ask the patient to take a deep breath and, as he exhales, ask him to say silently "relax and let go".

Instructions for relaxation: a relaxation session using Jacobson's technique is, typically, as follows:

"Keep your body loose and free, feet slightly apart, hands by side of body, palms up, slightly open" (Once the patient is in supine position, ask him if he needs to clarify anything. This helps develop confidence in the therapist as, generally, the patient is tense the first time).

"Close your eyes, direct your attention on your feeling within the body, keep the body calm, relax and feel the soothing sensation setting in."

FIST AND ARM

"Now clench the right fist, still more, a bit more, feel the tension within the palm, slowly release the palm, feel the tension leave the palm, feel the difference. Keep the body calm and relaxed." Repeat. Give similar instructions for the left fist. Repeat.

"Clench both fists simultaneously, tightly, a bit more, feel the tension in the palm, release slowly, feel the tension leaving your palm. Keep the body calm and relaxed." Repeat.

"Clench fists and bend the arms upwards, clench still more tightly, a bit more, feel the tension, release slowly, feel the tension leave, feel the soothing difference. Keep body relaxed and calm." Repeat.

"Keep your hands to the side, fan out your palms, stiffen the arm by clenching, feel the tension run through the arm, release slowly and surely, feel the difference." Repeat.

FACIAL MUSCLES

"Wrinkle your forehead upwards; still more, feel the tension, release slowly, feel the relaxed sensation, keep the body calm and relaxed". Repeat.

"Twitch your eyebrow, tightly, still more, feel the tension, release slowly, feel the difference, feel the calmness. Keep the body relaxed". Repeat.

"Close your eyes tightly, still more, feel the tension of your eyeballs, slowly release, feel the difference. Keep the body calm and relaxed." Repeat.

"Press the tongue to the roof of your mouth, still more, feel the tension, slowly release, feel the difference. Keep body calm and relaxed." Repeat.

"Open your mouth slightly and breathe slowly, clench your teeth, still more, feel tension in cheek muscles, release slowly, feels the difference. Keep body calm and relaxed." Repeat.

"Press your lips together, still more, a bit more, feel the tension, release slowly. Feel the soothing calmness. Keep body relaxed and calm." Repeat.

NECK MUSCLES

"Bend your head forward till chin touches chest, turn head to right, back to mid chest with chin touching chest. Now turn to left. Feel neck becoming light—come back to middle feel the tension being released." Repeat.

"Bend your head backwards with chin thrust upwards and tip of head on the couch. Turn right then return to middle position of head backwards. Turn left now and return." Repeat.

SHOULDER MUSCLES

"Bend your shoulders in an arc upwards slightly, feel the tension, release slowly by coming to normal supine position, feel the difference. Keep body calm and relaxed." Repeat.

"Press shoulders as much as possible into the couch. Feel the tensing of shoulder muscles, release slowly by coming to supine position. Feel the difference." Repeat.

"Move shoulders in a circular manner feel the tension while you do, slow down gradually, feel the difference. Relax and be calm." Repeat.

BACK BONE

"Bend the upper backbone, make it tight, as much as possible, release the tension slowly." Repeat.

"Bend the lower part of backbone, tighten it as much as possible, release slowly, feels the soothing sensation. Keep your body calm and relaxed." Repeat.

ABDOMINAL MUSCLES

"Swell your abdomen upward (while doing this breath through mouth). Feel the tension in your abdomen. Subside to normal position—and experience the tension leave. Be calm and relaxed." Repeat.

"Shrink your abdomen in, feel the tension as you shrink it in. Shrink it a bit more, release slowly." Repeat.

CHEST

"Draw in your breath and expand your chest and release slowly. Feel the difference between the two positions." Repeat.

THIGH MUSCLES

"Tighten your thigh muscles, feel the tension in the muscle. Gradually relax, feel the relaxation. Keep your body calm and relaxed." Repeat.

HEELS AND TOES

"Bend your heels down and feel the calf muscle tighten, bend the heels more and feel the calves tighten a bit more. Bring the heels to normal position feel the muscles relaxing." Repeat.

"Bend your toes in, towards the feet, feel the tension, release and bring toes back to normal. Bend toes back, feel the tension and bring back to normal. Feel the toes relax." Repeat.

After all muscle groups have been relaxed, give the following instructions:

"Let the muscles of your body relax slowly, remain loose and calm, draw in a deep breath and release slowly. Relax, relax…"

TERMINATION

Let the patient be in the supine position for ten more minutes, after which ask patient to count 1, 2, 3, 4 and 4, 3, 2, 1 after the therapist in a soft whisper. Ask him to open his eyes slowly. Gently ask patient to turn to one side (whichever side is more comfortable) ask patient to slowly get up and sit on the couch for a few seconds in a relaxed manner, and finally, ask him/her to get up from the couch.

IMPORTANT POINTS TO BE REMEMBERED

- All the sequences above have to be repeated twice, except when ending the session. Repetition helps in adaptation.
- While closing the fist, the thumb should be over the rest of the fingers.

- Opening of wrists etc. should not be too sudden or too slow, as the total efficacy may get affected.
- Extra care has to be taken while dealing with muscle relaxation. When pushing the upper backbone, the buttocks and the lower backbone should touch the couch.
- Do not let the patient just jump off from the couch. A slow and gradual manner is advisable as sudden jumping off may lead to blackouts and rise in blood pressure.
- Never let the patient go off to sleep except in case of insomnia, as sleeping further problems.
- Malingerers, patients suffering from hysterical disorders and patients with avoidance tendency etc., may sleep off half way through. In such cases, the therapist must be assertive and directive and wake up the patient.
- Usually in neurotic conditions, the patient learns to master the technique of relaxation by the eleventh session (barring obsessive-compulsive disorder patients and those in a highly tense state). In case of a more serious and willing patient, the time needed to master relaxation may be less.
- Relaxation is a self-controlled procedure to be done at least once a day, either in the early morning hours after ablutions, or after a day's work say around 5.30 in the evening. Relaxation done in the evening helps the patient sleep better.

CONTRAINDICATIONS OF RELAXATION PROCEDURES

- If patient has had a hernia operation or some major abdominal operation, the exercises should not be done
- Mental Retardation
- Children below 9 years
- Psychotics
- Old age and senility
- Epileptics with brain damage (Jacobson's relaxation is excellent with epileptics without brain damage)
- Suicidal patients (as relaxation depresses the functioning of cortex, the lower brain gets activated. This is responsible for emotional arousal. In the case of suicidal patients, this arousal may lead to bombardment of various ideas/thoughts which leads to strengthening of suicidal ideas and to consequent attempts that may be fatal)

- Relaxation Induced Anxiety (also known as the RIA Phenomenon): relaxation is generally done to put the individual in a state where he momentarily forgets his problems/worries and thinks more clearly. In some cases, it leads to an opposite result as in the RIA phenomenon wherein the individual ends up thinking more clearly about the stimulus which have actually caused him the problem and for which he sought help, further worsening the situation.

Jacobsons Differential Relaxation: is almost the same, except that after eleven sessions of Jacobson's progressive muscular relaxation Jacobson's differential relaxation comes into being. Here, only those muscles are relaxed which are enduring the stresses in the individual's life; in other words, relaxation is done only for the particular body part affected by stress.

Training in Imagery

Thoughts, images and mental activities can be both pleasant and unpleasant. The relaxation procedure requires that the patient's mind be trained to remain relaxed. Following this is the procedure called imagery training, in which the patient learns how to produce relaxing images and thoughts. Imagery training is used to block out intruding and upsetting ideas and its main goal is to reduce and control mental anxiety. Mental Imagery is like a daydream used to help the patient form images of pleasant things, including sensations of sound, touch and smell.

Steps in imagery training

Prepare by asking the patient to lie down or sit. Ask him to take a deep breath and exhale slowly, deeply and easily. As the patient takes the second breath and exhales, instruct him to imagine that he is floating and to experience the sensation of floating. As the patient does so instruct him to concentrate on the breathing, allowing it to become smooth and rhythmic. The therapist can, for example, start the imagery in the following manner:

(1) By asking patient to picture himself, standing on a mountain top where the weather is pleasant, the rain has stopped, and in the distance, is a white sandy beach dotted with green, swaying palm trees.

(2) Making the patient imagine that he is falling asleep under a tree, that he is beginning to dream and sees himself walking along a warm, sunny beach, at the edge of crystal clear water, hearing the roar of the waves. Suggest to the patient that he can feel the clean sand under his feet and smell the salty sea air.

(3) From here onwards, the therapist can help the patient move to a picture of himself sitting on a field of wild flowers on a spring day. Imagine that the temperature is right, the air is smelling of wild flowers and that he can hear soothing sounds of birds. In this way, help the patient to use his power of imagination to create a feeling of relaxation. Make the patient enjoy the feelings of relaxation and encourage him to stay in these for a while. Continue instructing the patient to breathe in and breathe out, enjoying the calming feeling of peaceful imagery. This allows the patient to control situation rather than be controlled by it.

(4) When the therapist wants the patient to come out of the imagery, he should count from 1 to 3, let the patient take a deep breath and then ask him to start counting 1, 2 and 3. As he reaches 3 ask him to open his eyes slowly and gently. The patient, at this point, will be alert and feel refreshed.

Systematic Desensitization

Systematic desensitization was developed by Lazarus and Wolpe who, through years of laborious experimentation, realized that systematic graded exposure to fear arousing stimuli combined with reciprocal ways to overcome the fears in gradual exposure can help render the patient asymptomatic.

Steps in systematic desensitization include:

Step I. Training in relaxation

Usually it takes eleven sessions for an average person to master technique of relaxation.

Step II. Construction of hierarchy

This is an important step in desensitization and is worked out with the help of the patient. A list of fear arousing or anxiety provoking situations is drawn up, starting from a neutral situation to the most anxiety or fear provoking situation. Then, the patient ranks the entire fear provoking or distressing situation from the least to the most or on a 10 or 15 point scale. For example, if the client suffers from a dog phobia, a possible listing could be as follows:

When standing very close to the dog, so close that it is:

Possible to reach out and touch him	→ Most distressing
The dog is loose, standing at the door of the same room	→ Ranked fourth
The dog is loose, in the next room	→ Ranked third
Can see the dog tied, at about 10 meters	→ Ranked second
Can hear the dog bark but not see him	→ Least fear arousing
A beautiful red rose	→ Neutral stimuli or situation

Construction of hierarchy is usually (*a*) monothematic (when the fear is one particular person, situation or thing) or (*b*) multi-thematic (when the patient fears more than one situation or thing). In this case, the therapist may develop two separate hierarchical lists and use them as required. (*c*) in terms of time, known as "temporal hierarchy". For instance if an individual has examination phobia, the list would be something on the following lines:

"Imagine yourself 3 months before the exam."
"Imagine yourself 1 month before the exam."
"Imagine yourself weeks before the exam."
"Imagine yourself 14 days before the exam."
"Imagine yourself 7 days before the exam."
"Imagine yourself 2 days before exam."
"Imagine yourself the morning before exam."

(*d*) Hierarchy can also be spatial that is, in terms of space. For example, if the individual suffers from dog phobia, then a spatial hierarchy list would be as follows:

"You are standing 15 meters from the tied dog."
"You are standing 10 meters from the tied dog."
"You are standing 5 meters from the tied dog."
"You are standing 1 meter from the tied dog."
"You are very close to the tied dog—you can reach out and touch him."

"You are petting him now."
"You have picked him up and are cuddling him and he is wagging his tail."

Step III. Starting desensitization

Once the patient has mastered relaxation and the hierarchy list prepared, the therapist begins with the process of desensitization based on the list prepared. He takes the least fear-arousing situation and instructs the patient to imagine it. The therapist also instructs the patient to raise the left index finger if he feels uneasy at any time and the right index finger if he feels no distress. When extremely tense, the patient is instructed to raise his hand. After giving instructions, pause for a minute before the next step.

Step IV

- Begin with neutral situation on the list—let the patient visualize it for 20 seconds.
- Instruct patient to feel calm and relaxed.
- Go on to the first distress arousing stimulus—let the patient visualize it for 20 seconds.
- Instruct patient to feel calm and relaxed.
- Carry on in this manner until the patient is completely relaxed while visualizing the distressing situation.
- Whenever the patient indicates to the therapist that he is uneasy, the therapist should stop and relax the patient immediately. When the patient is relaxed, allow him to remain that way for two minutes and then go on to the imagery of the neutral stimuli. For example, "visualize a beautiful red rose", give 20 seconds to visualize. Before the session is terminated, the patient should be completely relaxed.
- In the next session, the therapist should start all over again as above, until the patient is completely relaxed. As and when the patient feels uneasy, terminate the imagery, help the patient relax, go back to the neutral stimuli and on to the fear arousing stimuli. If the patient is unable to relax, then start the same procedure in the next session until the patient is able to overcome the distress in all the situations from the list prepared. Once the state of being relaxed

is achieved in the imagery of the most fear-arousing stimulus, give at least five to seven sessions of training to prevent any relapse.

Assisted Desensitization

This was developed to help those individuals who have difficulty in imagining and visualizing. This technique follows the same procedure of relaxation training and construction of hierarchy as in systematic desensitization. The difference here is that instead of asking the patient to visualize the various items in the hierarchy that are distressing, he is asked to talk about them. How the conversation takes place and how helpful it will be to the patient in the end depends largely on the therapist. As various every day items are presented, the patient is encouraged to talk about the fear-arousing stimulus. At all stages, the therapist pays close attention to whether the patient is feeling uneasy or not while talking of the various listed situations. If the patient feels uneasy, the procedure of relaxing him before continuing is followed. Thus, the procedure continues until the patient is able to talk about all the anxiety-provoking situations without feeling any distress.

Anger Management

Everyone experiences anger, which varies in its manifestation in different persons. While some when angry clam up, others shout or cry, and yet others destroy. Anger is a very common source of stress and can lead to disruption of important, interpersonal relationships, destruction of property and termination of occupation. Frustrations, total helplessness, unfair and unjust treatment or evaluation, being abused or attacked, being doubted on integrity might all lead to anger. Anger is an emotion that leads to aggression and violence, and causes irreparable damage to the individual as well as to those who are close to him.

Anger management is one of the important procedures to help a patient overcome aggressive behavior, depression as well as the negative consequences of the anger itself. The steps to be followed include:

Step I

The patient should be helped to look for tension that is building up in him, which prepares him to fight. The patient at this stage should be helped to identify the emotions and behaviors that are associated with his feeling angry.

Step II

The patient then is asked to note down the thoughts, ideas and situations that increase his anger and whenever he starts to feel tense, the patient is trained to give sub-vocal suggestion to himself, "my muscles are starting to feel a little tight, now is the time to relax, time to slow down". The patient should repeat this until he feels relaxed. In addition, he should be trained to repeat "my anger can remind me of what I need to do—it is time to help myself."

Step III

During this step, the patient is made to understand the need to be patient and listen to other point of view. For example, the patient is trained to say "let me take this issue step-by-step, may be the other person's point of view is also right. I do not lose anything by being co-operative."

Step IV

In this step, the patient is trained to consider the fact that his angry reaction may be due to the irrational belief that he needs to be perfect or right all the time. The patient is made to understand that it is a question of "what is right" and not of "who is right".

Step V

In this step, the patient is trained in the technique of how to deal with the anger-inducing person by making him run out of steam before starting the discussion. To relax while the other spends his steam—this is what the patient must learn to do. Then the patient is asked to make use of positive suggestions such as "He is trying to make me angry but I am going to disappoint him." Such statements help the patient to cope better with anger as and when it arises.

Step VI

This step consists of helping the patient deal with the anger caused by an insult or provocation when he is offguard. The patient is trained to handle anger in such situations by saying "The more I keep my cool the more I am in control." When someone insults him, it is important that he remember that he does not have to prove or defend himself but has to remain calm, cool and collected. The patient is taught to give positive suggestions to self. For example, "I do not need to prove myself" or "I do not need to doubt myself as I know who I am and what s/he says does not matter." This self-help talk helps the patient to focus on what he needs to do, rather than jumping to negative conclusions and getting angry over them.

Step VII

After the situation is over and the anger has passed, the patient is trained to learn to commend himself at having controlled the anger by his own efforts. Realizing and experiencing how he has coped successfully with his anger is the final step. The patient makes use of such statements as "I am doing better in this, I am pleased with my progress. Controlling myself was not as hard as I thought."

Step VIII

In this, many anger-provoking situations are role-played and the patient is trained to anticipate anger and take measures to control the same. For this, the therapist makes the patient generate an imagery of anger-provoking situations, has the patient experience anger, all methods are learned and rehearsed with the aim of controlling anger in different situations.

Assertiveness Training

There are three primary ways of communicating with others. These are: (*a*) Passive (*b*) Aggressive (*c*) Assertive.

Passive Behavior means that the person gives up his rights by not expressing his thoughts, honest feelings and beliefs. It often permits others to walk all over him. It can also mean that the person expresses himself in an apologetic way. A person can be considered behaving passively when he does what he is told, regardless of how he feels about it. Invariably, he feels helpless, anxious, resentful and, at times, even disappointed with himself. The goal of such passive behavior is usually to please others and avoid conflict or rejection. In contrast to this is *Aggressive Behavior*. Here the person stands up for his personal rights and expresses his thoughts and feelings in a way that is not helpful and usually affects the personal rights of others. An aggressive behavior may take the form of threatening, blaming and fighting, and these in turn cause the person to feel bitter, guilty or lonely afterwards. While the goal of passivity is to please others, the goal of aggressive behavior is to dominate, protect, vent, humiliate and force others to loose. Between these two extremes is *Assertive Behavior* which means that the person stands up for his personal rights, expressing his thoughts and beliefs in direct, honest and helpful ways, without violating the rights of others. Assertiveness means respecting oneself, expressing one's needs and defending one's rights as well as respecting the needs, feelings and rights of other people. Assertive behavior shows confidence, while, aggressive behavior aims at winning, assertive behavior does not guarantee a win, but definitely a compromise which makes others and the person himself happy.

Steps in assertiveness skills training

STEP I

Explain the different concepts of passive, aggressive and assertive behaviors to the patient by giving suitable examples. The therapist can give handouts of these behaviors which describe their verbal and nonverbal aspects. In the assertive form, such behavior includes (a) smiling when pleased (b) relaxed (c) no fidgeting (d) no slouching (e) good eye contact (f) not hostile (g) collaborative. The words and phrases used in such behavior include "I want", "I think", "I fear", "We could", "let us" and open ended questions like "How do you feel". *Passive behavior can be expressed through* (a) hunched shoulders (b) slugging (c) shifting body weight (d) whining (e) giggling or wringing hands (g) downcast eyes (h) quiet voice. Phrases and words include "may be", "I wonder if you could", "It is not important", "never mind". Aggressive behavior includes (a) leaning forward (b) pointing finger (c) thumping fist

(d) using a short, firm, sarcastic voice (e) dominating (f) shouting (g) violating the rights of others. Commonly used words and phrases are "your fault", "you had better", "you should, ought and must" etc.

STEP II

In order to assess the patient's needs correctly, the problem areas and the lack of assertiveness skills in different situations need to be identified. Some questions that the therapists could ask the patient include "Are you able to express positive/negative feelings", "Can you express a personal opinion", "Can you express justified anger or annoyance". In addition, the therapist should find out the situations in which the patient experiences problems in asserting himself. The patient should be given the questionnaire on assertiveness hierarchy and asked to complete it by ranking it in order of importance. A facsimile of assertiveness problem hierarchy is given below:

Assertiveness problem hierarchy form			
Name:			
Age:			
Date:			
Situations	High	Average	Low
Relationship with significant other (parent, sibling, spouse)			
Difficulty in taking criticism			
Feels guilty when saying "no"			
Unable to ask the superior for leave, when the need arises			
Unable to put one's viewpoint across to colleagues			
Unable to assert self with shopkeepers and others, when needed			

The patient is asked to indicate the problem with which he would like to start. Always start with the lowest rank problem and move to higher ranks.

STEP III

In this, the patient is asked to review the list of situations in which he has been passive, aggressive or assertive. He is also asked to record all his verbal and non-verbal behaviors in each situation. Following this, he writes down his goals for such behaviors. After reviewing what the patient is currently doing and his decision to become more assertive, the therapist helps him decide how he would like to handle the situation. He is then asked to write down a variety of responses that might be more effective than the current ones.

The typical tools used for training in assertiveness include the following:

BEHAVIORAL REHEARSAL

Here the patient is encouraged to rehearse the desired behavior. The therapist explores the problem chosen and, together with the patient, decides what the most suitable behavior for the given situation is. The therapist then demonstrates the behavior to the patient and asks him to practice it in his presence. To do so, the therapist takes the role of the person *vis-à-vis* whom the assertive behavior has to be exercised. The problems and difficulties that arise during the rehearsal are taken up and discussed in the therapeutic session.

MODELING

This is another method where the patient observes the therapist demonstrate a particular behavior before he practices it himself. Before demonstration, the therapist assesses whether the patient can actually perform that behavior and, only when he sure that he can, does he demonstrate and model it. The behavior that is to be learned is divided into easy-to-learn units. In the first unit, the patient is asked to try out one of the behaviors and the therapist gives his comments at the end of the exercise. This procedure is repeated a number of times. Home work assignments are given to the patient to practice, with easy situations to begin with and proceeding on to difficult ones. Whenever the patient experiences anxiety, he is asked to relax and when the levels of anxiety are reduced, the exercise continues. Modeling serves as a form of reassurance in graded exposures.

ROLE-PLAYING

This is another method by which the patient learns the skill that he wishes to acquire. He begins using the skills of assertiveness in a role-play situation that the therapist creates specially, in a group of three or four persons, each of whom takes up a role where the patient has to learn say to "no". At the end of the exercise, all the members of the group provide their comments and discuss the skills applied and the difficulties encountered.

VISUAL IMAGERY

In this method the patient imagines better ways of handling the problem. He is asked to take the role of someone who acts in an assertive manner—it is helpful to use a mirror to check the non-verbal messages. He is asked to take the role first of himself, then of the other person and, finally, his role again all the while imaging and rehearsing the possible outcomes.

PRACTICE SAYING "NO"

This helps the patient try out situations in which demands are made on him in his imagination and role-play them in front of the mirror.

FOGGING

This skill helps a person deal with criticism and "put-downs" and helps to protect self-esteem by acknowledging his mistakes.

WORKABLE COMPROMISE

Assuming one's self worth or self-respect is not being challenged, the patient offers the other person a workable compromise. Example: "You have to stay back and type this report, as it is needed at the head office." "I am afraid I have not made arrangements for child-care for the evening, but I could come in early tomorrow and complete the report."

References

Achenbach, T.M. (1991). *Youth Self-report for Ages 11–18*. Burlington: Dept. of Psychiatry, University of Vermont.

Andrasik, F., Turner, S.M., and Ollendick, T.H. (1980). Self-report and Physiologic Responding During In-vivo Flooding. *Behavioral Research and Therapy*, 18, pp. 593–95.

Badami, H. and Badami, C. (1988). Self-Analysis Questionnaire. In D.M. Pestonjee (ed). *Second Handbook of Psychological and Social Instruments*. New Delhi: Concept Publishing House.

Barrios, B.A. (1988). Behavioral Situations Test. In M. Hersen and A.S. Bellak (Eds.). *Dictionary of Behavioral Assessment Techniques* (pp. 69–72). New York: Pergamon.

Beck, A.T., Steer, R.A., and Garbin, M.G. (1988). Psychometric Properties of Beck Depression Inventory: Twenty-five Years of Evaluation. *Clinical Psychology Review*, 8, pp. 77–100.

Bellack, A.S. (1983). Recurrent problems in the behavioral assessment of social skills. *Behavioral Assessment*, 1, pp. 157–66.

Bellack, A.S. and Hersen, M. (Eds.) (1998). *Behavior Assessment: A Practical Handbook* (Fourth Edition). Boston: Allyn and Bacon.

Buck, J. (1966). *The House–Tree–Person Technique: The Revised Manual*. Los Angeles: Western Psychological Services.

Burns, R. and Kaufman (1970). *Kinetic Family Drawings*. Brunner Mazel: New York.

Charlesworth, E.A. and Nathan, Ronald (1984). *Stress Management—A Comprehensive Guide to Wellness*. Ballantine Books: New York.

Cooper, J. (1970). The Leyton Obsessional Inventory. *Psychological Medicine*, 1, pp. 48–64.

Derogatis, L. (1983). *Symptom Checklist 90-R Manual II*. Towson MD: Clinical Psychometric Research.

Diagnostic and Statistical Manual of Mental Disorders (Fourth edition) (1994). Washington DC: American Psychiatric Association.

Dryden, Windy (Ed.) (1996). *Handbook of Individual Therapy*. London: Sage Publications.

Dutt, N.K. (1966). Dutt Personality Inventory (DPI): Psychological and Educational Implication of the Concepts of Mental Health in Indian Thought. In Udai Pareek and T.V. Rao (1974). *Handbook of Psychological and Social Instruments*. Samashti: Baroda.

Eidelson, R.J. and Epstein, N. (1982). Cognitive and Relationship Maladjustment: Development of a Measure of Dysfunctional Relationship Beliefs. *Journal of Consulting and Clinical Psychology*, 50, pp. 715–20.

Eisler, R.M., Hersen, M., Miller, P.M., and Blanchard, E.B. (1975). Situational Determinants of Assertive Behaviors. *Journal of Consulting and Clinical Psychology*, 43, pp. 330–40.

Ellis, Albert and Harper, Robert (1961). *A New Guide to Rational Living*. California: Wilshire Book Company.

Erickson, E. (1980). *Identity and the Life Cycle*. New York: Norton.

Feldman, L.A. (1993). Distinguishing Depression and Anxiety from Self-reports: Evidence from Confirmatory Factor Analysis on Non-clinical and Clinical Samples. *Journal of Consulting and Clinical Psychology*, 4, pp. 631–38.

Gelder, M., Gath, D., Mayou, R., and Cowen, P. (1994). *Concise Oxford Textbook of Psychiatry*. USA: Oxford University Press.

Glass, C.R., Merluzzi, T.V., Biever, J.L., and Larsen, K. (1982). Cognitive Assessment of Social Anxiety: Development and Validation of a Self-Assessment Questionnaire. *Cognitive Therapy and Research*, 6, pp. 37–55.

Goodenough, F.L. (1926). *Measurement of Intelligence by Drawings*. New York: Harcourt, Brace & World.

Goodman, W.K., Price, L.M., Rasmussen, S.A., Mazure, C., Fleischmann, R.L., Hill, C.L., Heninnger, G.R., and Charney, D.S. (1989a). The Yale–Brown Obsessive-Compulsive Scale I: Development, Use and Reliability. *Archives of General Psychiatry*, 46, pp. 1006–11.

Goodman, W.K., Price, L.H., Rasmussen, S.A., Mazure, C., Delgado, P., Henninger, G.R. and Charney, D.S. (1989b). The Yale–Brown Obsessive-Compulsive Scale II: Validity. *Archives of General Psychiatry*, 46, pp. 1012–16.

Greenberger, Dennis and Christine A. Padesky (1995). *Mind Over Mood—A Cognitive Therapy Treatment Manual for Clients*. New York: Guilford Press.

Hallam, Richard (1992). *Counseling for Anxiety Problems*. London: Sage Publications.

Hammer, E.F. (1955). *The UFP Clinical Research Manual*. CA: Western Psychological Services.

Herzberger, S.D., Chan, E., and Katz, J. (1984). The Development of an Assertiveness Self-report Inventory. *Journal of Personality Assessment*, 48, pp. 317–23.

Heimberg, R.G., Chiauzzi, E.J., Becher, R.E., and Madrazo-Petersen, R. (1983). Cognitive Mediation of Assertive Behavior: An Analysis of the Self-statement Patterns of College Students, Psychiatric Patients and Normal Adults. *Cognitive Therapy and Research*, 7, pp. 455–64.

Hodgson, R.J. and Rachman, S. (1977). Obsessional-Compulsive Complaints. *Behavior Research and Therapy*, 15, pp. 389–95.

Hollon, S.D. and Kendall, P.C. (1980). Cognitive Self-Statements in Depression: Development of an Automatic Thoughts Questionnaire. *Cognitive Therapy & Research*, 4, pp. 383–95.

Ivnik, R.J., Malec, J.F., Smith, G.E., Tangalos, E.G., Peterson, R.C., Kokmen, E., and Kurland, L.T. (1992). Mayo's Older Americans Normative Studies: WAIS-R Norms for ages 56–79. *Clinical Neuropsychologist*, 6 (suppl.), pp. 1–30.

Jones, R.G. (1968). A Factored Measure of Ellis Irrational Belief System with Personality and Adjustment Correlates. Unpublished Doctoral dissertation. Texas Technical College. USA.

Kapur, Malavika (1995). *Mental Health of Indian Children*. New Delhi: Sage Publications.

Kaplan, H.L., Sadock, B.J., and Grebb, J.A. (1994). *Synopsis of Psychiatry* (Seventh Edition). New Delhi: B.J. Waverly Private Ltd.

Kazdin, A.E. (1974). Self-monitoring and Behavior Change. In M.J. Mahoney and C.E. Thoresen (Eds.). *Self Control: Power to the Person*. Monterey: Brooks/Cole.

Kerlinger, F. (1973). *Foundations of Behavioral Research* (Second Edition). New York: Rinehart and Winston.

Kirk, J. (1989). Cognitive Behavioral Assessment. In K. Hawton, P.M. Salkovskis, J. Kirk and D.M. Clark (Eds.). *Cognitive Behavior Theraphy for Psychiatric Problems: A Practical Guide*. Oxford : Oxford Medical Publications, pp. 13–51.

Koskal, F. and Power, K.G. (1990). Four Systems of Anxiety Questionnaire (FSAQ): A Self-report Measure of Somatic, Cognitive Behavioral and Feeling Components. *Journal of Personality Assessment*, 54, pp. 534–45.

Lemma, A. (1996). *Introduction to Psychopathology*. London: Sage Publications.

Levenson, R.W. and Gottman, J.M. (1978). Towards the Assessment of Social Competence. *Journal of Consulting & Clinical Psychology*, 46, pp. 453–62.

Lewinsohn, P.M. (1974a). A Behavioral Approach to Depression. In R.J. Freedman and M.M. Katz (Eds.). *The Psychology of Depression: Contemporary Theory and Research*. New York: Wiley.

——— (1974b). Clinical and Theoretical Aspects of Depression. In K.S. Calhoun, H.E. Adams and K.M. Mitchell (Eds.). *Innovative Treatment—Methods of Psychopathology*. New York: Wiley.

Lovibond, S.H. and Lovibond, P.F. (1992). Self-report Scales (DASS) for the Differentiation and Measurement of Depression, Anxiety and Stress. Cited in A.S. Bellack and M. Hersen (1998). *Behavioral Assessment—A Practical Handbook* (Fourth Edition). MA: Allyn & Bacon.

Mandler, G. and Sarason, S.B. (1952). A Study of Anxiety and Learning. *Journal of Abnormal and Social Psychology*, 47, pp. 166–73.

Marks, I.M., Hallam, R.S., Connelly, J., and Philpott, R. (1977). *Nursing in Behavioral Psychotherapy*. London: Royal College of Nursing of the United Kingdom.

Marks, I.M. and Mathews, A.M. (1979). Brief Standard Self-rating Scale for Phobic Patients. *Behavior Research and Therapy*, 17, pp. 263–67.

Mattick, R.P. and Peters, L. (1988). Treatment of Severe Social Phobia: Effects of Guided Exposure with and without Cognitive Restructuring. *Journal of Consulting and Clinical Psychology*, 56, pp. 251–60.

McGlynn, F.D. and Rose, M.P. (1998). Assessment of Anxiety and Fear. In A.S. Bellack and M. Hersen (Eds.). *Behavioral Assessment—A Practical Handbook*. Allyn & Bacon, Boston. USA.

Mehrotra, L.P. (1992). *TAT Manual: Indian Adaptation*. New Delhi: Psycom Services.

Mersch, P.P.A., Emmelkemp, P.M.G., Bogels, S.M., and Van Der Sleen, J. (1989). Individual Response Patterns and the Effects of Behavioral and Cognitive Interventions. *Behavior Research and Therapy*, 27, pp. 421–34.

Meyer, T.J., Miller, M.L., Metzger, R.L., and Borkovec, T.D. (1990). Development and Validation of Penn State Worry Questionnaire. *Behavior Research and Therapy*, 27, pp. 421–34.

Moreno, J.L. (1945). *Psychodrama*. New York: Beacon House.

Murray, H.A. (1943). *Manual of Thematic Apperception Test*. Cambridge, MA: Harvard University Press.

Palmer, S. and Dryden, W. (1995). *Counseling for Stress Problems*. London: Sage Publications.

Pareek, Udai and Rao, T.V. (1974). *Handbook of Psychological and Social Instruments*. Baroda: Samashti.

Patel, A.S. (1956). Anxiety Index Scale: A Rationale, Construction and Try-Out of Test Scales Measuring Some Personality Traits. *Advances in Education*, 1 (2), pp. 11–27.

Pestonjee, D.M. (Ed.) (1988). *Second Handbook of Psychological and Social Instruments*. New Delhi: Concept Publishing Company.

Raj, J. Bharath (1992). *Manual for Medico-Psychological Questionnaire*. Mysore: Swayamsiddha Prakashana.

Riggs, D.S. and Foad, E.B. (1993). Obsessive-Compulsive Disorder. In D.H. Barlow (Ed.). *Clinical Handbook of Psychological Disorders* (Second edition). New York: Guilford.

Roberts, L.J. and Leonard, K.E. (1992). Intimacy Avoidance and Conflict Avoidance in Early Marriage: Predictors of Relationship Satisfaction. Paper presented at the 26th Annual Convention of the Association for the Advancement of Behavior Therapy. Boston.

Rorschach, H. (1951). *Psychodiagnostics: A Diagnostic Test Based on Perception*. Tr. by P. Lewkall and B. Kronenberg. New York: Grune & Stratton.

Rotter, J.B. and Rafferty, J.E. (1950). *The Rotter Incomplete Sentences Blank: College Form*. New York: The Psychological Corporation.

Salzman, L. (1995). *Treatment of Obsessive and Compulsive Behaviors*. Northvale, N.J.: Jason Aronsen.

Sanders, Diana (1996). *Counseling for Psychosomatic Problems*. London: Sage Publications.

Sinha, D. (1968). *Sinha's Anxiety Scale: Manual for Sinha W–A Self-Analysis Form in Hindi*. Varanasi: Psychological Corporation.

Skodol, A.E. (1987). *Problems in Differential Diagnosis, From DSMIII TO DSMIII-R in Clinical Practice*, USA: American Psychiatric Press. Inc.

Spielberger, C.D. (1972). Anxiety as an Emotional State. In C.D. Spielberger (Ed.). *Anxiety: Current Trends in Theory and Research*. New York: Wiley.

Spielberger, C., Gorsuch, R., Lushene, R., Vagg, P., and Jacobs, G. (1983). *Manual for the State–Trait Anxiety Inventory*. Palo Alto, CA: Consulting Psychologists Press.

Srivastava, D.N. and Tiwari, G. (1973). *The Anxiety Scale*. Agra: Agra Psychological Research Cell.

Stewart, R.L. and Levin, M. (1967). Psychotherapies. In A.M. Friedman, H.I. Kaplan and H.S. Kaplan. *Textbook of Psychiatry*. New York: Williams & Wilkins.

Straus, M.A. (1979). Measuring Intrafamily Conflict and Violence: the Conflict Tactics (CT) Scales. *Journal of Marriage and the Family*, 41, pp. 75–88.

St. Lawrence, J.S., Kirksey, W.A., and Moore, T., (1983). External Validity of Role-play Assessment of Assertive Behavior. *Journal of Behavioral Assessment*, 5, pp. 25–34.

Teri, L. and Lewisohn, P.M. (1982). Modification of the Pleasant and Unpleasant Events Schedule for Use with the Elderly. *Journal of Counselling and Clinical Psychology*, 50, pp. 444–45.

Thorpe, G.L. and Olson, S.L. (1990). *Behavior Therapy: Concepts, Procedures and Applications*. USA: Allyn & Bacon.

Turner, S.M., Beidel, D.C., Dancu, C.V., and Stanley, M.A. (1989). An Empirically Derived Inventory to Measure Social Fears and Anxiety: The Social Phobia Anxiety Inventory. *Psychological Assessment*, I, pp. 35–40.

Verma, S.K., Wig, N.N., and Preshad, D. (1985). *Manual for PGI Health Questionnaire N-1*. Agra: National Psychological Corporation.

Walk, R.D. (1956). Self-ratings of Fear in Fear-invoking Situation. *Journal of Abnormal and Social Psychology*, 52, pp. 171–78.

Watson, D. and Friend, R. (1969). Measurement of Social Evaluative Anxiety. *Journal of Consulting and Clinical Psychology*, 33, pp. 448–57.

Watson, D., Clark, L.A., and Tellegen A. (1988). Development and Validation of Brief Measures of Positive and Negative Affect: The PANAS Scales. *Journal of Personality and Social Psychology*, 54, pp. 1063–70.

Wilson, P.H., Spence, S.H., and Kavanagh, D.J. (1989). *Cognitive Behavioral Interviewing for Adult Disorders: A Practical Handbook*. UK: Routledge.

Wolpe, J. and Lang, P.J. (1964). A Fear Survey Schedule for Use in Behavior Therapy. *Behavior Research and Therapy*, 2, pp. 27–30.

Wolpe, J. and Lazarus, A.A. (1966). *Behavior Therapy Techniques: A Guide to the Treatment of Neurosis*. New York: Pergamon.

Wolpe, J. (1973). *The Practice of Behavior Therapy* (Second edition). New York: Pergamon.

Index

About the Authors

Vimala Veeraraghavan is currently a Professor at the Department of Applied Psychology, University of Delhi (South Campus). Prior to this she was Associate Professor, Zakir Hussain Centre for Educational Studies, Jawaharlal Nehru University; and Assistant Professor, Department of Social Work, Delhi University. She has also been a Visiting Professor at Thammassant University, Bangkok, Thailand. Professor Veeraraghavan has had a distinguished career spanning more than three decades in the fields of mental health, counseling, education, and research in areas like drug abuse.

A specialist in the clinical and counseling areas, she is a well-known practitioner in addition to being a consultant to numerous international and national organizations dealing with mental health issues and is a member of various apex bodies at the national and state levels. Professor Veeraraghavan has not only published eight books so far but has also contributed chapters in books as well as numerous articles to reputed journals. She has served as the Editor-in-chief of the *Behavioural Medicine Journal*.

Shalini Singh is currently a Lecturer at the Department of Applied Psychology, University of Delhi, (South Campus). A specialist in clinical psychology, Dr Singh has extensive experience in counseling and in conducting workshops for teenagers and adolescents. She has also worked with an NGO on issues of HIV/AIDS and sexuality. Shalini Singh has presented papers in various conferences and is also the co-author of *Teenage Blues* and *HIV/AIDS: An Interdisciplinary Approach to Prevention* and *Management*.